Three know truths about preventing and treating cancer.

First, 80% of all cancers are associated with environmental causes like smoking, chewing tobacco, alcohol, radiation, and drugs.

Second, there are some well known signals of cancer which must be recognized and investigated.

Third, most cancers, when detected and treated early, are curable.

Medical science today has the capability and technology to control, and largely prevent, cancer. However, we need to overcome our fear and any tendency to procrastinate — both can be fatal.

This book seeks to inform. It deals with some well-recognized causes of cancer; lists signs and symptoms that we must learn to recognize; explains investigations that may be required; and discusses methods of treatments and of disease management.

Prevention, awareness and early detection are the objectives that bind the book together without confusing the reader with unnecessary medical jargon.

The Author

Prof. Dr. O.P. Jaggi is a medical scientist of international standing. He is the former Dean of the faculty of Medical Sciences, University of Delhi, and Director of V. Patel Chest Institute, Delhi

He firmly believes in the concept of preventive medicine and, therefore, in explaining medical facts. he has written and spoken extensively on health and medicine, both in India and abroad. His books on healthcare including *Asthma & Allergies; Prevention and Treatment; Asthma in Children; Healing Systems and You Can Prevent Heart Attack* have been immensely popular. His deep commitment to patient care has won him wide recognition.

He can be contacted at Asthma, Chest and Allergy Centre, 128, Vasant Enclave, New Delhi-110 057.

Cancer

Prevention and Treatment

Dr O P Jaggi
MD, PhD, FCCP (USA)
FACA (USA), FRAS (LON)

Orient Paperbacks
DELHI | MUMBAI

Disclaimer

This book has been designed to provide information and to educate. The authors and Orient Paperbacks shall have neither liability nor responsibility to any person or entity with respect to any loss, damage, or injury caused or alleged to be caused directly or indirectly by the information in this book. The information presented herein is in no way intended to subsitute or replace medical counselling.

www.orientpaperbacks.in

ISBN: 978-81-222-0062-1

1st Published 1990
19th Printing 2025

Cancer: Prevention & Treatment

Cover design by Vision Studio

Published by
Orient Paperbacks
(A division of Vision Books Pvt. Ltd.)
5A/8 Ansari Road, New Delhi-110 002

Printed and bound at Saurabh Printers, Noida.

Preface

Cancer, as a disease, has existed all along with man. Hippocrates, twenty-five centuries ago, called it ***karkinois*** because the swollen blood vessels going and coming from the tumour mass, gave the appearance of the claws of a crab. Susruta described cancer as a tumour which would ulcerate and would not cure and "sow its seeds in other parts of the body".

Knowledge about cancer has been gradually gathered over the centuries. Incidence of cancer is increasing in most parts of the world. Cancer being more common in older people, increasing life span of man is providing more and more candidates for getting the disease.

Smoking of cigarettes, air pollution and increasing use of chemicals, pesticides in particular which in one form or another enter our bodies, act as direct causes of cancer.

Surgery to treat it has been used since centuries ago. Radiation was used to treat breast cancer within one year of Roentgen's discovery World War Two, provided the first drug in the form of nitrogen mustard to kill cancer cells.

In the 1950s, only 30 per cent cancers were curable. By 1977, that percentage had risen to 41. By 1980, 45 per cent of all serious cancers were curable; this percentage is increasing fast.

More important than cure is the prevention of cancer. We know that 80 per cent of all cancers are associated with environmental causes: smoking, chewing tobacco, dietary substances, alcohol consumption, radiation, work-place substance exposure, drugs, etc.

Fighting cancer is not just hoping to discover a "magic bullet" to annihilate it. It is much broader a problem: early detection, curative measures, rehabilitation of the patient, psychological problems faced by a patient and his relatives

Remarkable strides have been made in fighting cancer during the last two decades. The author feels that spreading knowledge is itself a step towards fighting cancer.

Contents

Investigation of Liver:
- Biochemical Tests
- Isotope Scan
- Ultrasound Scan
- CT Scan
- Liver Biopsy

Investigation of Pancreas:
- Biochemical Tests
- Ultrasound and CT Scans

Investigation of Gall-Bladder:
- Oral Cholecystogram
- Intravenous Cholangiography
- Endoscopic Retrograde Cholangiopancreatography (ERCP)

Investigation of the Lungs:
- Bronchoscopy
- Laryngoscopy
- Pelural Biopsy and Aspirate
- Lung Functions Tests
- Lung Scans

Investigation of Kidneys:
- Intravenous Pyelogram (IVP)
- CT Scan
- Isotope Scan
- Ultrasound Scan
- Renal Biopsy

Investigation of Nervous System:
- Lumber Puncture and Myelogram
- Ultrasound and CT Scan

Investigation of Cervix of the Uterus:
- Pap Smear Test
- Biopsy of the Cervix

Investigation of the Thyroid:
- Thyroid Scan
- Fine Needle Aspiration Biopsy

Investigation of a Lymph Node
- Biopsy Examination
- Lymphangiogram

1

What is Cancer?

All living things such as germs, insects, animals and human beings are made of numerous cells. Human body itself is made up of millions of cells that are specially adapted to carry out particular functions—such as the sex cells, sperms and ova, carry out the functions of reproduction.

Now, what is a cell? The cell is the basic unit of all living things or organisms, which can reproduce itself exactly. A collection or mass of cells of one kind is called tissue—such as nervous tissue, muscular tissue, connective tissue, etc. And aggregation or collection of tissues constitutes organs, such as heart, lungs, liver, etc. In other words, an organ is a part of the body, composed of more than one tissue.

As the human body grows from infancy to adulthood, the cells belonging to different tissues and organs divide and subdivide until no more increase of the cells is required except for the normal wear and tear of the body. Normally the rate at which an organ should grow and when it should stop growing, is under the control of the body itself.

Cancer arises from the abnormal and uncontrolled division of cells, known as cancer cells, that then invade and destroy the surrounding tissues. Cancer cells, in other words, refuse to stop multiplying and continue to increase in number. It is the failure to stop multiplying which is the hallmark of cancer. This they do even at the cost of other normal cells of the body which are starved to death for lack of nutrition.

Cancer cells are different from normal cells in some aspects. They do not remain confined to one part of the body. They penetrate and infiltrate into the adjoining tissues and dislocate their function. Some of the cancer cells get detached from the main mass or site of origin and travel by blood and lymph channels to sites distant from the original tumour and form fresh colonies, called metastasis or secondary growths, in other organs where they grow at the cost of the normal cells. This is how they destroy the well-regulated functioning of the body and bring about its end.

A cancer may be slow-growing or fast-growing. The rate at which a cancer grows depends on the tissue in which it occurs and also on the inherent character of the type of cancer. Rapidly-growing cancers are those which send metastasis in other organs, are much more dangerous. Sometimes the primary cancer in first stage of development grows slowly, as for example, that of the stomach and remains unnoticed, while the secondaries spread rapidly in the liver, abdominal lymph glands, etc. These secondary cancers are first noticed.

Growth of cancer cells leads, generally, to formation of a nodule or tumour. Hence, cancer is also called a tumour. If it is superficial, it is firm to touch, gets fixed to surrounding tissues and is not freely moveable. Every nodule, however, is not a cancer. Some like warts, cysts, or adenomas are benign and are easily treated. But in order to be sure whether a nodule is cancerous, a bit of the nodule is taken and examined under the microscope. This generally gives a correct diagnosis.

How Does Cancer Spread?

One of the biggest problems with cancer is its spread in different parts of the body. This spread occurs through any or all of the three following routes:

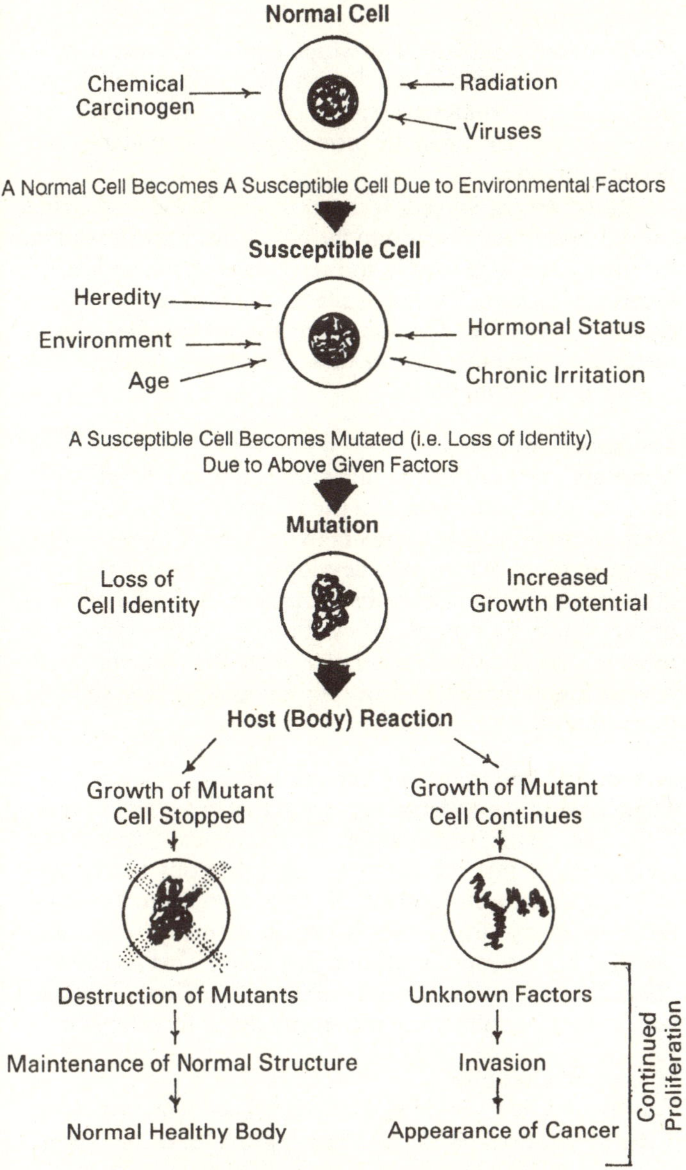

Causes & Gowth of Cancer Cells in Humans

Local Spread: The cancer infiltrates the adjoining parts, organs, tissues, etc.

Lymphatic Spread: The lymph glands or nodes trap the cancer cells present in the lymph fluid and cancer grows within them. Progressive spread along lymph vessels and glands may occur and in the process quite distant glands may become involved.

Bloodstream Spread: If cancer invades blood vessels then the cancer cells may break into the bloodstream and be carried to other parts of the body and settle over there, producing secondary cancers. The major site of spread in cases of bowel cancer is the liver. The lungs are the commonest site of metastasis from other cancers sites. The spread to many other organs is also common.

Is Cancer Inherited?

There are cases of some families, several members of which have suffered from cancer. In the laboratory, scientists have been able to propagate some strains or breed of mice in which a large number of the males developed lung cancer and over 90 per cent of the females breast cancer. A careful analysis of data shows that certain types of cancer are hereditary and there is a likelihood of cancer of a particular tissue or organ developing in the descendants of persons who have suffered from cancer.

Is Cancer Contagious or Infectious?

There is so far no evidence to suggest that any kind of cancer in human beings is contagious or infectious. Experiments conducted in this regard by taking cancerous tissues and injecting or implanting them on human volunteers once or twice or many times, over a period of many weeks and months, has not produced cancer in them. This shows that normal people have some defence mechanism in their bodies which does not allow the cancerous tissue to take root.

Is Cancer Curable?

Cancer is curable, provided it is detected and removed before it has penetrated into other adjoining tissues or has spread through metastasis to other organs of the body.

Remarkable progress has also been made during the past two decades in the treatment of cancer by the use of surgery and radiation therapy. The discovery of a variety of anti-cancer drugs have, to a large extent, revolutionised the treatment of cancer during the past few years.

Types of Cancer

Carcinoma: Any cancer that arises in epithelium, the tissue that lines the skin and internal organs of the body.

Sarcoma: Any cancer of connective tissue. These tumours may occur in any part of the body, as they arise in the tissues that make up an organ rather than being restricted to a particular organ. They can arise in fibrous tissue, muscle, fat, bone, cartilage, blood and lymphatic vessels, etc.

Leukaemia: It is a cancer of the blood in which the bone marrow and other blood forming organs over-produce immature or abnormal white cells.

Lymphoma: Any malignant tumour of lymph nodes or lymph gland.

Signs and Symptoms of Cancer

Cancers of various types and at various sites manifest

Any of the following manifestations may be cancer:

1. A lump or hard area in the breast.
2. A change in a wart or mole.
3. A persistent change in digestive and bowel habits, for example, constipation.
4. A persistent cough or hoarseness in a smoker.
5. Bleeding per vagina at times other than the menstrual.
6. Non-injury bleeding from the surface of the skin, mouth of any other bodily orifice.
7. Any ulcer that does not get well.
8. Unexplained loss of weight.
9. Unexplained diminished or lost appetite.
10. Unexplained low-grade fever.

themselves in a variety of ways.

On external surfaces, any thickening of the tissues, formation of a nodule or tumour, persisting sores and ulcers, can be a feature of cancer.

Internal cancers may grow for some time before they cause any symptom. But weight loss, anaemia and low-grade fever in older people even without any other symptom, should arouse suspicion.

Cancer in Children

Some cancers occur more often in children. The following table shows their type and the percentage of the total cancers in childhood.

Type	% of Total Cancers
Leukaemia	30
Nervous system (Retinoblastoma)	12
Bone sarcoma	12
Soft tissue sarcoma	12
Neuroblastoma	10
Wilms' (kidney) tumour	8
Lymphoma	8
Hodgkin's disease	6
Others	2

Cancer in Older People

Cancer occurs more often in people after 50 or 60 years of age. In still older people, i.e. 80 years or above, some characteristics of cancer have been noted during life and in post-mortem studies of people who have died of causes other than cancers.

1. Small microscopic cancers of the prostate were very common in males.
2. Lung and stomach cancer were seen in many cases, both in males and females.
3. Lung cancer of the type of adenocarcinoma, was

found often and was commoner in females than males.

4. Multiple cancers arising in different organs at the same time was not an uncommon feature.
5. Lesions regarded as precursors to cancers were often observed in stomach, colon and lungs.
6. The rate of growth of cancers in general was slow.

Cancer Situation in the World

Cancer is the second common cause of death in the developed countries next to cardiovascular (heart and blood vessel) diseases. In Europe and North America, approximately one in five die of cancer. According to WHO, out of an estimated total of 50 million deaths annually in the world, more than 5 million are attributed to cancer, and the number of deaths from cancer throughout the world is increasing.

Cancer Situation in India

Approximately 500,000 new cases of cancer occur every year in India. As the human life span is increasing in India, more cases of cancer are observed here also. Cancer is thus regarded as an emerging health problem in India. According to Dr. D.J. Jussawalla, founder secretary of Indian Cancer Society, "Cancer is one of the 10 leading causes of death today in India, and is advancing in rank year by year."

The figures given by Indian Cancer Society state that about 1.5 million people suffer from cancer at any point of time in India. Oral cancer and Cervix cancer account for the major causes of cancer in this country.

2

Some Well-Recognised Causes of Cancer

As in any other disease, in cancer also, both the environmental as well as the genetic factors, play a role in the causation of the disease. Over the last few decades, it has been found that the environment plays a prominent role in the causation of most cancers. 80 to 90 per cent of all cancers are said to be dependant directly or indirectly on environmental factors. Cancer problem in the world and in India is fast increasing with the increasing industrialisation and the presence of innumerable chemicals and fumes in the environment, changes in life-style including smoking and eating habits.

Environmental Factors

Among the environmental factors that can cause cancer, the following are the well-recognised ones.

Physical Reagents or Reactive Substances

In the England of the eighteenth century, naked boys used to crawl down chimneys to sweep them before the beginning of winter. Many of these boys, as they grew up, were noticed to develop cancer of the scrotum, i.e. the sac that holds the testes and the skin over the abdomen. The cause of this cancer was found to be the deposition and rubbing of soot, coal-dust and coal tar on their skin over many years. Later on, scientists isolated from coal tar, substances such as dibenzanthracene, which could cause skin cancers in mice when it was painted daily on their skins for a period of a few months.

Benz(a) pyrene, a substance akin to dibenzanthracene has been seen in a number of edibles and in the environments, including places of work. The distribution of benz(a) pyrene in nature is very wide, as smoke contains the substance along with other polycyclic aromatic hydrocarbons, and during rains these are brought down to the earth, where in turn, these are taken up by the vegetables and plants.

Numerous other chemical agents have either been identified or come under suspicion. The list is a long one: tars, dyes, aromatic amines, urethane, various metals, e.g. nickle, beryllium, arsenic, chromium, asbestos, hormones, and more recently aflatoxin.

A number of chemicals utilized as medicinal compounds can cause cancer. Diethyl stilbesterol (female sex hormone) is probably the best example having been shown to cross the placenta and cause vaginal cancer (adenocarcinoma) in offspring of women who have taken large doses during their pregnancy. The use of estrogens (female sex hormones) in menopausal women has also been found to be associated with a very significant increase in risk of uterine cancer.

Alkylating agents and other compounds employed in the treatment of cancer are carcinogenic, i.e. can cause cancer, in animals and their potential risk as well as risk benefit considerations must be carefully evaluated.

Mesothelioma, a cancer of the pleura, a covering layer over the lungs, is a rare tumour, occuring in individuals exposed to asbestos. In recent years, it has been found that asbestos workers also have a significantly increased risk for lung cancer. Here again, however, this risk is associated with smoking which has a dramatic synergistic effect. The asbestos worker who is also a heavy smoker has a 20-fold increase in risk of lung cancer. Cancer of the urinary bladder has been found to occur frequently in workers in aniline dye (synthetic colour) factories.

Thus, we see that there are many cancer-causing chemicals in our environment, exposure to which for longer or shorter duration, can make one liable to getting lung and other cancers.

Smoking Can Cause Lung Cancer

The suspicion that cancer of the mouth is somehow associated with the use of tobacco goes as far back as 1739 AD. In the nineteenth century, several cases of cancer of the mouth were reported in which chewing of tobacco was incriminated.

A correlation between increase of cigarette smoking and the rising incidence of lung cancer was, for the first time, commented upon during the first quarter of the twentieth century, in the USA, Germany and Great Britain. It was, however, only in 1950's that a cause-and-effect relationship could be shown to exist, with a fair certainty between excessive cigarette smoking and the development of lung cancer. This came about as a result of intensive clinical and epidemiological, as well as experimental studies the world over.

Clinical Studies: More than thirty such studies have been conducted so far in ten countries including Great Britain, USA, West Germany, Finland, France, Japan, the Netherlands, Norway and Switzerland. The British investigations, started in 1947 under Dr. Doll and Dr. Hill, drew the maximum attention. This inquiry covered 1465 lung cancer patients who were compared with an equally large group of carefully selected controls (those of same age and sex but not having cancer). The analysis of the data from this and other studies revealed the following facts:

1. Smokers run a greater risk of getting lung cancer.
2. This risk increases with the greater amount of tobacco consumed; heavy smokers (more than 25 cigarettes a day) run a much higher risk.

In another study carried out in Britain, a questionnaire

was sent in 1951, to 60,000 doctors of or above the age of 35 years. Sufficient information was received from 40,000 of them to enable the investigators to classify the smokers according to the prevailing smoking habits at the time of enquiry. Upon the death of any of them, the necessary details as regards the causes of death were obtained and confirmed. The results obtained were as follows:

Lung cancer mortality increases consistently and steeply with increased tobacco smoking. For heavy smokers (25 gm or more a day), the mortality is 24 times more compared to non-smokers, for moderate smokers (15-24 gm a day), it is 12 times more, and for mild smokers (1-14 gm a day), it is seven times more.

The American follow-up studies of Dr. Hammond and Dr. Horn, took into consideration the smoking habits of 187,766 male whites between the ages of 50 and 70 years belonging not only to large and small towns but also to rural areas. Their conclusions were:

Those who regularly smoke up to 20 cigarettes a day are about 25 times more prone to lung cancer than a non-smoker; this figure mounts to roughly 45 times for those who smoke between 20 and 40 cigarettes a day and reaches a multiple of approximately 90 for chain-smokers who smoke more than 40 cigarettes a day.

Besides the above studies, there are other interesting observations which indicate the cause-and-effect relationship between cigarette smoking and lung cancer.

1. In Iceland, the people smoked very little until after 1941, when they took to it because of the contacts offered by the American occupying troops. An analysis of the post-mortem examinations performed between 1932 and 1938, revealed lung carcinoma to be a rare disease.

2. On post-mortem examination of 11,365 pairs of lungs of Bantu miners in South Africa who died between 1916 and 1949, lung cancer was found only in 6 cases, while it was found 114 times more among 8465 white miners. Bantu people scarcely smoked cigarettes, white population did.

3. A much higher death rate from lung cancer was found

among European-born Jews in Israel in 1957, than among those born in Asia and Africa; in the latter countries, during the preceding decades, cigarettes were not so popular.

4. In a non-smoking, non-drinking community of the Seventh Day Adventists in the United States, between 1952 and 1956, only one case of lung cancer was observed, and if we take into consideration the general population, there should have been at least 10 to 11 cases of lung cancer.

5. Lung cancer has scarcely been seen among the Sikhs in India; they are, by their religion, forbidden to smoke or use tobacco in any form.

6. Examination of lungs of smokers dying from causes other than lung cancer has revealed a step-by-step change in the lung cells leading towards lung cancer.

Animal Experiments: Tobacco tar obtained after distillation of tobacco and the same applied on the shaved skin of the mice for some weeks, produced in the skins of only some animals the cancerous changes.

Later, when smoke tar collected under conditions simulating human smoking, and the same was applied on the shaved skin of mice, and the process continued for about their natural life span, changes in the skin somewhat related to lung cancer in human beings, were detected.

When mice were exposed to tobacco smoke in glass vessels and the process was continued for weeks on end, some changes suggestive of leading towards lung cancer could be produced in some.

Experiments were carried out under simulating conditions akin to human smoking. For example, a batch of 24 dogs was taught to inhale smoke by means of tubes inserted directly from their wind pipes into the lungs. Two and a half years later, after having smoked seven cigarettes a day, two of these animals developed lung cancer similar to those of human beings.

Many smokers, by now, know that smoking causes lung cancer, but somehow think, "Its not likely to happen to me". A victim of such fallacy was one of the eminent doctors, a member of the ten-man commission appointed in 1962, by

US Surgeon-General to study and to advise the Government on the health hazards of smoking. While he, with his colleagues, clearly found and stated that cigarette smoking causes lung cancer, he, a chronic smoker, continued smoking. At the age of 66, even though he had cough and breathlessness on exertion, he considered himself in good shape to take up a new assignment. A routine medical check-up, however, revealed a small mass in his lung which on further examination was declared to be lung cancer. Fortunately for him, it was detected at a very early stage, and was removed by operation. He was saved. But in the majority of the smokers who get lung cancer, it is detected and diagnosed at a stage where operation is not possible because of its spread in the surrounding organs or its metastasis in far off organs. The initial symptoms of lung cancer in smokers are not very much different from the usual cough and breathlessness which they may have had for years.

I cannot forget a person whom I had known years before as a man of athletic built, handsome, and with a face radiating life. He came to my clinic, some time ago, and I could hardly recognize him: face pale and puffy, breathless as he entered the room, his finger nails looked to me almost white because of anaemia. His relatives laid before me a bundle of X-rays. It was a case of advanced lung cancer. I thought, he will live at the most, two more months. Later I was informed, that he survived only six weeks. He was 47 then and had been a chronic smoker since the age of 18.

Tobacco and its Smoke: Tobacco smoke is a gas mixture containing finely divided solid and liquid particles. Under the electron-microscope the major portion of it is found to consist of liquid droplets in the shape of an aerosol. This smoke is said to contain in it about a thousand chemical constituents, of which approximately 270 have been recognized already. The important among them are the nicotine, carbon monoxide gas and a mixture of many chemicals which form, on deposition, a brownish tarry substance commonly called smoke tar.

The active agents in the tar which lead to the production

of cancers have been identified as different polycyclic aromatic hydrocarbon compounds.

These are not present initially in the tobacco but are produced as a result of incomplete combustion of tobacco. Roughly about 20 mg of smoke tar passes inside the body of the smoker when he smokes one cigarette. A person who smokes 20 cigarettes a day, thus absorbs about 150 gm of smoke tar in a year. Judging from the effect of its application on laboratory animals, it seems an immense amount to be able to cause serious damage in the lungs.

X-Rays, Radioactive Substances and Solar Radiation and Cancer

During the nineteenth century, among the mine workers of the Schneeberg and Jachymov mines, now in Czechoslovakia, cases of lung cancer were detected in greater frequency than in the surrounding areas. It was later found out that these mines contained various radioactive substances which were the cause of cancer.

Experimentally also, prolonged exposure of laboratory animals to X-ray or other radioactive substances has been shown to produce cancer. Many inexperienced technicians working with X-ray machines in the past, were found to develop cancer of the skin over the hands and even developed leukaemia commonly called 'blood cancer'. Bone cancers were noted to have occurred more frequently in girls who were engaged in watch factories to paint dials of watches with luminous paint which contained radioactive material. Leukaemia and other cancers have been shown to have occurred among many Japanese who were exposed to the atom bomb explosions.

Solar radiation has its share in the causation of cancer. In Australia, New Zealand and some parts of the USA, skin cancers are common and this is attributed to the adverse effect of sun's rays.

Chronic Irritation Can Cause Cancer

A slight but constant injury over a period of many years, has been known to lead to cancer of that part of the body. A jagged edge of a broken tooth rubbing against the tongue, gall stones rubbing constantly against the gall-bladder, the smoking short clay pipes used by labourers in Europe, have led to cancers of tongue, gall-bladder, and the lips, respectively. In the Godavari region of Andhra Pradesh, many men and women smoke locally rolled cigars (*chutta*) with the burning end inside the mouth. Some of these people are known to develop cancer of the mouth. *Kangri* cancer among the Kashmiris develops over the skin of abdomen and thigh. This is due to the constant injury by the hot *kangri,* which is an earthen pot containing burning coal kept underneath the garments directly in contact with the skin. The dhoti cancer below umblicus seen among Maharashtrian men and women has been attributed to chronic irritation leading to cancer.

Some Viruses Can Also Cause Cancer

Many cancers in animals, plants and birds have been recognized to be caused by viruses. Currently, it is being convincingly stated that leukaemia and Hodgkin's disease—i.e. a malignant disease of lymphatic tissue—are associated with some kind of virus.

Association of Hepatitis-B virus with primary liver cancer is now fairly well established. The African lymphoma described by Burkitt in 1958, is suspected to be due to Epstein-Barr virus.

Although in 1911, Peyton Rous first showed that a virus caused sarcoma in chickens, it was not until the late 1950's and early 1960's with the isolation of the murine (mice) leukaemia viruses and the discovery of the polyoma virus, that serious consideration was given to a virus etiology or cause for human cancer and great expectations for control with vaccines were generated.

When these viruses enter the cells they are supposed to upset the normal chemical reaction inside the cells which leads to mutation of these cells into cancer cells.

Hormones and Cancer

Cancer of the prostate in men and of the breast in women can be greatly relieved by the removal of the testes and ovaries, respectively, in these patients, or by the removal of adrenal glands which are a secondary source of sex hormones in both sexes. Besides this, administration of counter-hormones (estrogens in males and androgens in females) in such cases also effects a marked improvement.

Environmental factors described above do not lead to cancer in all those exposed to them. So it seems, that something is there in the person to make him susceptible to getting it.

Genetic and Personal Factors

Among the genetic and personal factors age, sex, race, marital status, etc. have much to do about the prevalence of cancer.

Age

The prevalence of cancer increases with age. Man is particularly vulnerable after the age of 50. It is not certain whether this is due to a) the changes in the body due to the ageing process, b) a long incubation period of cancer or c) long exposure to a carcinogen or cancer causing substance.

Sex

There are sex differences in the frequency of cancer, e.g. lung cancer and cancer of the oesophagus are more common in men than in women.

Race

The influence of race is difficult to disentangle from that of environment. Fair-complexioned individuals have an excessive frequency of cancer of the skin especially of the face and neck than coloured races.

Marital Status

Cancer cervix is more common among the married and among those who marry at an early age.

Heredity

Genetic influences have long been suspected. Napolean is said to have died of cancer of stomach; his grandfather, father, brothers and sisters, all died of cancer of stomach. Retinoblastoma, i.e. cancer of the eye occurs in the children of the same parents. Osteosarcoma or malignant cancer of the bone, polyposis colon or cancer of colon and thyroid cancers in twins, are other examples. It is recognised that mongols are more likely to develop cancer or 'blood cancer' (leukaemia) than normal children. There are strong indications that chromosomal damage and deformity is characteristic of some forms of cancers, but a definite cause-effect relationship has not been established.

Socio-economic Status

There is a definite relationship between socio-economic status and cancer frequency. For example, cancer of stomach, skin and cervix are more common in low income than in high income groups. Breast cancer is commoner among women of higher socio-economic group, probably because of late child-bearing.

Immune Defficiency Can Cause Cancer

Transformation of normal cells into cancer cells in the body, is not a rare event. But the body's defence or immunologic cells—lymphocytes and macrophages—at once recognise these abnormal cells and kill them before they get divided and subdivided into many more.

In a person exposed to carcinogenic or cancer causing agents, this transformation of normal cells into cancer cells occurs more often and some of the cancer cells do not get killed in time and so are able to set up a cancer.

Moreover, an immune deficient person exposed to carcinogenic agents the normal surveillance provided by the defence immunologic cells is weakened, so that not all cancer cells get killed and those which remain, are in a position to set up the disease.

3

Tips for Early Detection of Cancer

Early detection of cancer is vital to its successful treatment. In order to do so, there are some symptoms and some risk factors which if present in a patient should arouse the suspicion of the disease. He should then consult urgently his physician or a specialist. The symptoms and risk factors are as follows:

Symptoms

Bleeding: Bleeding after slight injury; vomit mixed with blood; non-injury bleeding from the surface of the skin, mouth or any other bodily orifice or opening; blood in the stool; bleeding per vagina other than menstrual one or after the sexual act or vaginal discharge mixed with blood; phlegm containing blood: blood in urine, continued bleeding after delivery; bleeding from a mole or what looks like a mole, etc.

A Lump or Hard Area: Lump in the abdomen which is found out to be the spleen; a lump in the thyroid; a lump in the inner lining of the lip; lump in the neck; a lump or nodule in the breast; a lump in the muscle; a lump in the arm; a lump in the leg, etc.

Raised Birthmark: Sudden growth in a mole, or

birthmark; bleeding from a mole, or what it looks like a mole; formation of a new moles, around an old one, etc.

A Hardbase Chronic Sore That Does Not Heal: Particularly if located on the penis or inside of the penis that covers the glans.

Constipation: More so if alternating with loose motions.

Pain and Tender Swelling of the Bone and the Tissue Around it: It may involve bone to break it without much of an injury; continuous and increasing pain over a bone, etc.

Loss of Weight: Weight loss without any visible cause especially among adults, in spite of good appetite and intake of nourishing food items.

Diminished Appetite: Diminished appetite or loss of appetite and aversion to taking food.

Feeling of Tiredness: It may be without any apparent reason or accompanied by low-grade fever and increasing weakness, and anaemia.

Painless/Painful Swellings: It is different from nodular swellings or a lump—such swellings can be often on one side of the neck or the abdomen; painless swelling with a hard base in the cheek; discomfort or pain sometimes severe in the upper abdomen; enlarged and painful testes, etc.

Difficulty in Swallowing: Difficulty in swallowing solid or semi-solid food or vomiting of food that has been taken lately, sometimes mixed with blood.

Risk Factors

Smoking: Those who have been smoking for more than 20 years.

Tobacco Chewing: Those who have been chewing tobacco for more than 15 years.

Industrial/Vehicular Pollution: Those who are over-exposed to vehicular pollution or working or staying around industrial townships/areas.

Asbestos: Those who are exposed to asbestos in asbestos manufacturing workshop.

Exposure to Frequent X-rays: Those who are exposed to frequent X-rays for investigations or those who are working in any capacity in the X-ray departments.

Oral Contraceptives: Women consuming pills, etc. for years by way of mouth for avoiding pregnancy.

Different Sexual Partners: Women having sexual relations with multiple or different partners.

Menopause: Women who have attained the stage of menopause are susceptible to uterine cervix cancer. After menopause they should regularly undergo investigation for uterine cancer.

Early Marriage and Frequent Pregnancies: One should undergo investigation for suspected uterine cancer after the age of 40.

The symptoms and risk-factors out lined above can raise the suspicion of cancer. The next chapter gives details about all the investigations that may be needed to convert the suspicion into a confirmed diagnosis.

4

Investigations that may be Required for Cancer Check-up

In order to find out whether a person is suffering from cancer or not, one may not have to go to the doctor for investigations. The doctor may proceed as follows:

1. History taking
2. Physical examination
3. Laboratory investigations

However, a doctor may either proceed through all the three steps or he may be able to arrive at a diagnosis only through history taking and physical examination. One should leave it to the doctor for proceeding with the investigations.

History Taking

The aim is to get from the patient an accurate account of his complaints: how the symptoms started, how they progressed, what treatment the patient took and with what results. This information is recorded under the following heads:

Presenting complaints
History of present illness
History of past illness
Family history of any disease
Social and personal history of the patient, e.g. whether he is a smoker

Occupational history
Treatment history

History taking is as much a science as it is an art. The important thing is for the doctor to make the patient comfortable and at ease so that he narrates all that the doctor needs to know. Social and personal history of the patient as well as the occupational history are important aspects when cancer is suspected.

Physical Examination

After having taken the complete history, the doctor does the physical examination of the patient. This includes the general examination of the body, and the local examination of the part from which the complaints of the patient arise.

The important points that are noted are general appearance of the patient, i.e. whether the patient looks well or unwell, properly nourished or malnourished, has or has not lost weight, looks depressed or anxious, has pain or not, etc. Besides these the following points are also to be noted:

Pulse rate
Temperature
Blood pressure
Breath rate
Any swelling anywhere in the body
Wasting of any part of the body

Certain examination are also important, such as:

Examination of the throat, nose, eyes, ears, neck
Examination of the abdomen
Examination of the heart
Examination of the chest
Examination of the nervous system
Examination of the skin, nails, bones, muscles and limbs.
Examination of the genitals in males, including the rectal examination for the prostate glands, and examination of the female genital parts which includes examination of the vagina and the cervix of the uterus.

General Laboratory Investigations

There are whole lot of laboratory investigations to aid quick and definite diagnosis. But one may not have to undergo all these tests and investigations.

It is for the doctor to suggest investigations that may be required for a particular person suspected of cancer of a particular part or area of the body. The investigations may be general in nature or related to cover specific organ system.

Urine

Urine passed into a clean vessel is suitable for routine urine testing. Special methods of collection designed to reduce contamination are desirable for microscopic examination, and essential for bacteriological examination. The urine should be examined physically, chemically, microscopically and bacteriologically.

Naked Eye Examination: Quantity, colour, transparency, specific gravity, naked-eye characteristics of the deposits, are noted. The normal quantity of urine passed daily varies widely from 700 to 2500 ml, depending on the fluid intake and the weather.

Chemical Examination: Many of the traditional chemical tests for urinary constituents have been replaced for routine purposes by commercial tablets or reagent stick or strip tests.

Commonly tested biochemicals in urine are sugar and albumin; others are blood derivatives such as bile pigments and ketones.

Microscopic Examination: Urine is centrifuged at 1000-1500 rpm for ten minutes and the deposits examined microscopically. Red blood cells, white blood cells, epithelial cells, crystals and bacteria are looked for and reported.

Bacteriological Examination: A midstream urine specimen is collected after the vulva or glans penis has been cleaned with tap-water. It is suitable for most bacteriological purposes. Antiseptic solutions are not used for cleaning, as they may kill the bacteria present in the urine.

The most satisfactory specimen for cultures or tests is the one collected first after arising from sleep, because bacteria in the bladder have been able to multiply undisturbed for several hours. Presence of many bacteria in the urine indicates an infection.

Faeces (Stool)

No patient with bowel disturbance has been properly examined until the stool has been inspected. The white surface of a bed-pan makes an ideal background for the detection of blood, pus and mucus.

Naked Eye Examination: The following points are noted:

Amount
Colour
Odour
Form and consistency
Abnormal ingredients

Chemical Examination: Tests for altered blood is done.

Microscopic Examination: This examination is done to look for ova or cyst of the different worms that infest the intestines.

Examination of Blood

Routine examinations carried out on blood are :

Haemoglobin (Hb)
Red blood cell count (RBC)
White blood cell count (WBC)
Differential white blood cell count (DLC)
Erythrocyte sedimentation rate (ESR)

Other investigations are:

Platelet count
Bleeding time
Clotting time
Blood group

Examination of the Sputum

Sputum in patients may be purulent, containing pus or blood in it. It may be foul smelling.

Microscopic Examination: The principal value of microscopic examination of the sputum is in the detection of bacteria and recognition of cancer cells in cases of cancer of the lungs. Skill is required to differentiate cancer cells from the epithelium and other cellular debris.

X-Rays and Imaging

X-ray films are taken of the part of the body under investigation. Some dense tissues like bones, absorb more of these X-rays than others such as the lungs. As a result, in the X-ray picture of the part, we see some areas white indicating more density and some areas dark, indicating less density. Knowledge of how a normal structure looks like, helps in finding out where the fault lies in the X-ray picture of the patient.

X-ray examination involves exposure of a part of the body to X-rays. This should not be done in a pregnant woman. X-ray examination can be divided into two categories:

a) Plain
b) With contrast

Plain X-ray films are taken without any prior preparation. Usual X-rays of the chest and bones, etc. fall under this category. Removal of the clothing which may obstruct the X-rays partly or wholly, is necessary.

Contrast films are taken when a particular hollow organ, like intestines, urinary or gall-bladder or blood vessels are to be delineated.

Tomogram: The usual plain X-ray, as for example, of the chest, shows in one plane, all the structures present from back to front, and it becomes difficult to gaze the exact situation of the abnormality.

Tomogram is a series of X-rays taken at different distances from the back, for example, 3 cm, 7 cm, 10 cm, 15 cm or 20 cm or so. This helps in seeing and placing the abnormality more sharply, for follow up or for surgical operation.

CT Scan: It is computerized tomogram, also called CAT scan (computerized axial tomography). In CT scanning, the

X-ray source rotates round the part of the body under examination, and the X-ray detector receives information of the density of the body at a particular point of the body. When the scanner and the detector have rotated around the body, the information obtained from all angles is processed by a computer, which produces a picture on the television screen, showing the density of all the body's structures in the area about which it has rotated. This picture is of a slice of the body as thin as 1/2 cm or more, as required. An X-ray record of each slice can be taken, and thus a composite picture emerges.

Herein we have plain X-ray, not of the part of the body collectively seen from back to front (posterior to anterior), but a slice of the body part under examination. We can see that part, just as we see the section of a thin potato wafer. We can visualize the slices of the body, one after the other, so that we can estimate the extent of the lesion and its exact location.

The usual tomogram shows less resolution, so that the visibility of the part is poor. But in CT scan, the visualization is very clear.

Radioisotope Tests: A very small quantity of a particular radioactive material is injected intravenously in a patient. This particular material has the property to get concentrated in a particular organ, as for example, radioactive iodine in thyroid. The total quantity of radioactivity and its dimension in an organ is scanned by a camera called gamma camera. This tells whether the whole or part of the organ has taken the radioactive material and also whether the organ has taken more or less than the normal, thereby indicating the disease affecting the organ.

Ultrasonic Tests: Sound waves of very high frequency which a human ear cannot hear from a fine source called the 'probe' are pressed against a part of the body through which they pass and strike internal organs of various densities and are then bounced back and recorded. This record compared with the normal, gives an indication of the size of an organ or part of an organ and any abnormality indicated therefrom.

This can be seen on the television screen and recorded on an X-ray film. No special preparation is necessary and it causes no discomfort or after effect to the patient.

Biopsy Examination

Although a doctor may suspect cancer, a diagnosis cannot be established without examining a piece of the suspicious tissue under the microscope.

If the cancer is situated on the surface of the body, taking biopsy is easy. If, however, it is situated inside the body, then the surgeon has to open up the overlying part, reach in and then take the biopsy.

Biopsy can also be taken by passing a lighted tube in a hollow organ, (endoscope). When it reaches the involved organ, a piece of the involved tissue is taken with the help of a needle or a punch, coming from inside the endoscope. The piece of tissue taken is then processed and examined under the microscope.

Cancer-markers in the Blood

Cancer cells differ from normal cells histologically. The biochemicals they produce and pour in the blood are also different. The presence of cancer tissue in the body, may be detectable by the presence in the blood of biochemical products known as cancer or tumour-markers. These are normal metabolic constituents that are found either in abnormal amounts or at an inappropriate time of life, for example, foetal proteins being re-expressed in adult life. Tumour-markers of this type are useful in making diagnosis of some cancers. The presence of a tumour-marker can also be of clinical value in monitoring the progress of individual patients known to have a particular cancer.

Specific Laboratory Investigation of System/Organ

Investigation of Gastro-intestinal Tract

Examination of the Vomit: The character of the vomit varies with the nature of the food ingested and the absence or presence of bile, blood or intestinal obstruction. In obstruction of the stomach at the distal end, i.e. farthest from the stomach (pyloric stenosis), the vomit is apt to be copious and sour smelling, contains recognisable food eaten many hours before and exhibits froth on the surface. In case of an ulcer in the stomach, if the bleeding is much, the colour of blood in the vomit is red, but if the bleeding is less, then it gets altered to dark brown colour like coffee by contact with gastric juice. If there is obstruction in the intestine, the vomit may smell and look like faecal matter.

Examination of Ascitic Fluid: If the patient has swollen abdomen and physical examination reveals presence of fluid, then this fluid is removed either for diagnostic or for therapeutic purposes, in order to relieve him of the discomfort. The fluid withdrawn is sent for cytological, bacteriological examination and chemical analysis.

Barium Meal: A contrast meal such as barium compound, opaque to X-rays is given to the patient to swallow. This makes the part opaque in contrast to the rest of the structures, so that any abnormality such as a filling defect can be noticed on the X-ray.

Stomach cancer shows on X-ray as a filling defect in the barium-filled organ. The whole examination requires 6 to 24 hours to complete. Patient is asked to take light meal the previous night and not to take anything in the morning till the X-ray examination is over.

Barium Enema: Light food, preferably with least residue is taken for two days before the test. No solid food is taken the night before the test. A laxative is given a day before the test. An enema is done to wash the lower bowel clean.

Barium mixture is run into the bowel by a tube inserted into the rectum above the anus. The barium is seen by the radiologist on the X-ray screen in the dark room and wherever necessary, he takes the X-ray. The barium is then evacuated and further films taken.

By this means, obstruction to the colon in the large intestine by cancer and other abnormalities can be detected.

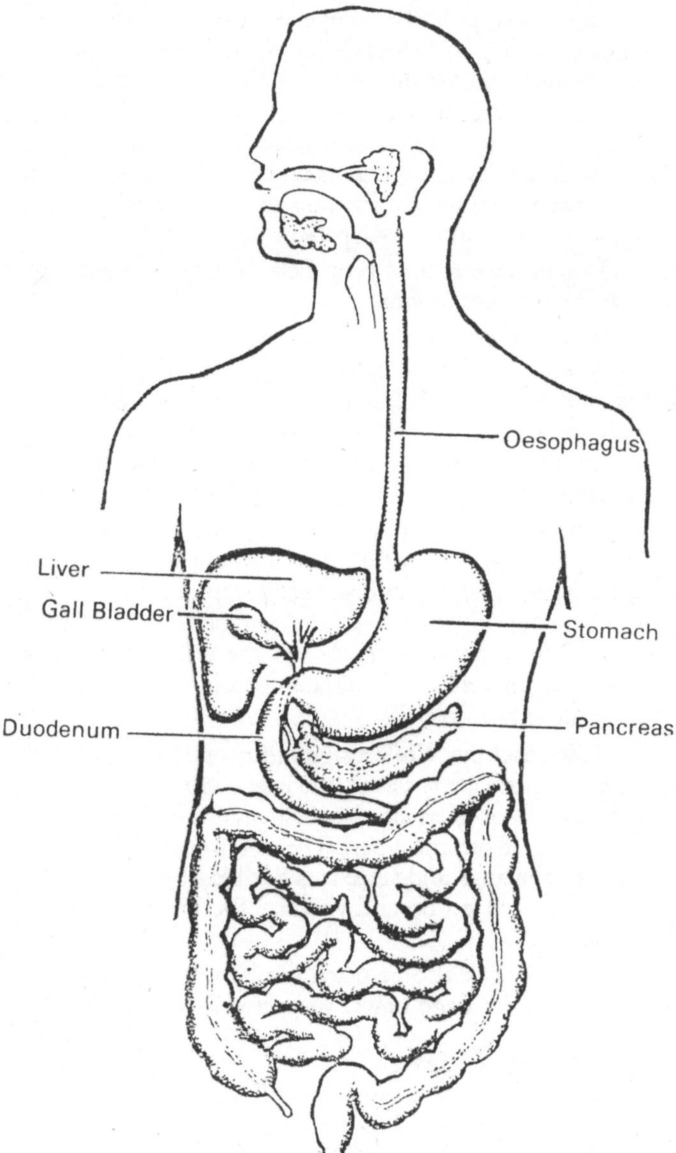

Gastro-intestinal Tract

Gastroscopy: A gastroscope, made up of a bundle of fibre glass, is flexible. It is introduced through the anaesthetized mouth and pharynx into the oesophagus, the stomach and up to the duodenum. With its front and side source of light, it can see all structures that it passes through directly. Also wherever necessary, it can take a punch biopsy which is examined histologically and a diagnosis made of the disease. It can be done in the out-patient department.

This procedure is of great help in differentiating cancer from non-cancer lesions.

Proctoscopy: The anal canal and lower rectum can be readily seen with a proctoscope. The patient cleans his bowels first, if there is urge. He is placed on the bed in a side position with knees bent. The lubricated instrument is passed to its full length. The lower end of the gastro-intestinal tract is seen directly.

Sigmoidoscopy: It is often necessary to examine the rectum and colon more fully than is possible by proctoscopy, and in such cases sigmoidoscope is employed. A lubricated stainless steel tube with small light bulb at the front, is inserted into the anus gently and the walls of the rectum examined for cancer or any abnormality. It causes only a discomfort but no pain.

Colonoscopy: While a sigmoidoscope is a metallic hard tube, colonoscope is elastic, the inside of which is made up of a bundle of glass fibres which transmit light from the source to its front-most part. The colonoscope is introduced through the anus and since it is flexible, it can bend round the curves and go up and visualize the whole of the large colon.

A biopsy can also be taken through the colonoscope of the part of the large bowel suspected of any disease.

Investigation of Liver

There are many tests to assess liver function and to know the nature of its disease.

Biochemical Tests: These tests are used in :

1. Differential diagnosis of jaundice
2. To detect liver cell damage in other disorders, and
3. To monitor the results of surgery of the biliary system and pancreas. These include urinary urobilin, plasma bilirubin, alkaline phosphatase, a serum aminotransferases, plasma proteins, plasma prothrombin and sulphobromophthalein excretion test, etc.

Isotope Scan: The radioactive material injected intravenouly is particularly concentrated in the liver, and can be seen on the television by the gamma camera and also be photographed. The abnormal part of the liver does not take it up and thus shows absence of activity over there. The test takes about one hour to complete.

Liver cancers and other diseases can thus be detected and demarcated by this procedure.

Ultrasound Scan: A probe emitting ultrasonic pulses is passed across the liver and surrounding areas. Echoes detected from within the patient are received amplified and suitably displayed.

CT Scan: Computerized tomography can be used to produce cross-sectional images of the liver, and is of value in detecting and demarcating lesions over there.

Liver Biopsy: This is taken by inserting a special needle through the anaesthesized skin over the liver area on the right side of the upper abdomen. The patient is asked to breathe out and then to hold the breath, so that when the needle is in the liver, it is not moving about with respiration.

Blood of the patient is tested before the biopsy is taken in order to see that there is no bleeding tendency in the patient and no risk of bleeding from the liver puncture site.

The piece of liver taken into the hollow needle or the liver cells present in it, are spread on a glass slide, fixed, stained and examined for histological picture and diagnosis of the disease.

Investigation of Pancreas

Biochemical Tests: Pancreas is a compound gland, about

15 cm long, that lies behind the stomach. Examination of the secretions of the pancreas can give an idea about cancer of the pancreas. For this purpose, a special double-lumen tube is swallowed and then screened into position in the duodenum, i.e. the first of the three parts of the small intestine. It has a weighted bulbous end and contains two sets of holes, one for duodenal and the other for gastric aspiration. The latter set of holes prevents contamination of the duodenal fluid that is aspirated.

After a short period allowed for stabilization, pancreozymin is injected and the duodenal aspirate collected for 30 minutes. The volume of aspirate and concentration and output of bicarbonate, amylase, lipase and trypsin are then measured and calculated. Patients with cancer of the pancreas produce low volumes and concentration of enzymes.

Fresh aspirate is examined for cancer cells by the Papanicoloau method. Interpretation, however, is difficult and requires an experienced cytologist.

Ultrasound and CT Scans: These are both useful methods in the diagnosis of pancreatic disease. Each method can differentiate solid from cystic lesion greater than 2.5 cm in size and the success rate in diagnosis is around 70 per cent.

Investigation of Gall-bladder

The main functions of the gall-bladder are to concentrate and store bile that is produced in the liver and to empty it into the duodenum after appropriate stimuli.

Oral Cholecystogram: The organ is investigated by performing oral cholecystography. This procedure depends on the fact that certain iodine-containing compounds, when absorbed in the gastrointestinal tract, are excreted by liver and concentrated in the gall-bladder, thus rendering it opaque.

A contrast mixture is taken by mouth which appears in the gall-bladder. An X-ray taken of the gall-bladder reveals its outline as well as any abnormality, including stones in it or any narrowing or obstruction due to any cause. It usually takes about two hours to complete the test.

Intravenous Cholangiography: It is used to demonstrate the bile ducts. The technique depends on the fact that an intravenously administered, iodine-containing compound is excreted by the liver in the bile in such a concentration that it is radio-opaque, i.e. opaque to X-ray and, therefore, does not depend on the concentrating power of the gall-bladder, as in cholecystography.

ERCP (Endoscopic Retrograde Cholangiopancreatography): This examination is done to visualize the ducts of the gall-bladder and the pancreas.

The flexible gastroscope is entered into the duodenum and there, the ducts of the gall-bladder and the pancreatic openings are recognised. A fine catheter (plastic tube) is passed down the gastroscope and into one of the ducts. When the catheter is in the duct, which is visualized on television screen, a small quantity of the radio-opaque dye is injected into the duct to be investigated, and its outline seen and X-rayed to assess whether there is any obstruction in it or not.

This test requires a very skilled gastroscopist. The patient is not put to much discomfort and the test is over in about an hour.

Investigation of the Lungs

Bronchoscopy: This is done for looking directly at the larynx, trachea, the two main bronchi and their subdivisions. Two types of bronchoscopes are used—the rigid and the flexible. Both have their uses, but the procedure with the flexible one is easy.

The bronchoscope is introduced generally through one of the nostrils, past the pharynx, the vocal cords, into the larynx, trachea and bronchi. The nostrils, the pharynx and the larynx are locally anasthetized with a spray anaesthetizer.

The bronchoscope has arrangement for seeing the parts directly. It also has a hollow narrow tube in it, through which secretions in the airways can be sucked out. A wire with an arrangement for taking punch biopsy as well as taking a smear with a brush from the suspected surface of the airways are also there.

The procedure is helpful for making a diagnosis of lung cancer, it can also see whether the vocal cords are working properly or not; this examination is usually done in cases of hoarseness of voice. There may be a cancer of the vocal cords in the larynx which if detected early, can be removed surgically.

Laryngoscopy: A small round mirror, a rupee-coin size is inserted in the mouth and pharynx, with the tongue held out, the mirror reaches the back (posterior) wall of the pharynx from where the shadow of the larynx and vocal cords in the mirror can be seen by the doctor doing this test.

Pleural Biopsy and Aspirate: If fluid collects in the pleural space around the lungs and is seen to be present in the X-ray films, then a small quantity of this fluid is removed by inserting a needle through the skin into the pleural space.

Whatever cause has led to the presence of the fluid in the pleural cavity, has its effect on the pleural surfaces also. So if a piece of the inner pleural surface is removed and examined histologically, it shows cause of the disease, whether it be tuberculosis or a cancer.

For taking this piece of pleura, a special needle is used, which after insertion punches out the required piece. While this is being done, the patient holds breath, so that there is no movement in the lung or the pleura due to breathing and a tear in it does not occur.

Slight pain or discomfort does occur at the time of taking the biopsy. In some cases, some air may also collect in the pleural space, the process called pneumothorax, but this air disappears usually in a day or so.

Lung Function Tests: These are helpful in the following circumstances:

1. To get an objective assessment of the patient's disability of the lungs.
2. To follow the progress of a disease and the effect of treatment.

3. To try to differentiate the possible causes of patient's breathlessness.
4. To assess patients prior to anaesthesia and surgery, particularly thoratic surgery leading to lung resection or surgical removal of lung.

Lung Scans: The lung is scanned:

1. To see the flow of blood in the blood vessels (perfusion).
2. To see the air in the lung (ventilation).

For perfusion scanning, i.e. for scanning the passage of blood through the lung capillaries the isotope is injected intravenously, and for ventilation scanning, the air that the patient breathes is mixed with a radioactive gas so that wherever that air goes, it can be seen and recorded by the gamma camera. Perfusion scan is done to see any abnormality or block in the blood vessel, such as is the case in pulmonary embolism in which a blood clot is carried in the circulation to lodge in the pulmonary artery and thus obstructs the blood flow. Ventilation scan is done to see in which part of the lung, the air does not go or come back, as happens in cases of emphysema, i.e. condition of enlarged or damaged air sacs (alveoli) of the lungs.

Investigation of Kidneys

Intravenous Pyelogram (IVP): This is done to outline the two kidneys, the bladder and the two ureters that connect the kidneys with the ureters.

In order to do this, not only is the contrast needed to fill these organs, but the whole of the intestine needs to be cleared and cleaned so that, their shadow does not mask the picture of the urinary tract.

Patient takes laxatives for two days before the test so as to clean the intestines. The liquid contrast medium is injected into the vein at the forearm. Mixed with the blood, this material appears first in the kidneys, then the ureters and then the bladder. A series of X-rays are taken of the abdomen, starting 5 minutes after the injection and up to one hour.

These X-rays reveal the outline of the kidneys, ureters and the bladder, and also tell the abnormality or obstruction in its parts.

CT Scan: The kidneys are easily examined in radiographic slices of the body, produced by computed X-ray tomography.

Isotope Scan: The special isotope is injected into the vein, and scanning done over the kidney, which reveals any abnormality that may be present in it. It may take about two hours to complete the test.

Ultrasound Scan: The kidneys and their gross structure are relatively easily demonstrated by ultrasound examination.

Renal Biopsy: By means of a special needle inserted from the back, biopsy is taken from the kidney and examined histologically. Considerable skill is required. There is a small but definite risk to the patient.

Renal biopsy examination clinches the diagnosis of the disease he is suffering from.

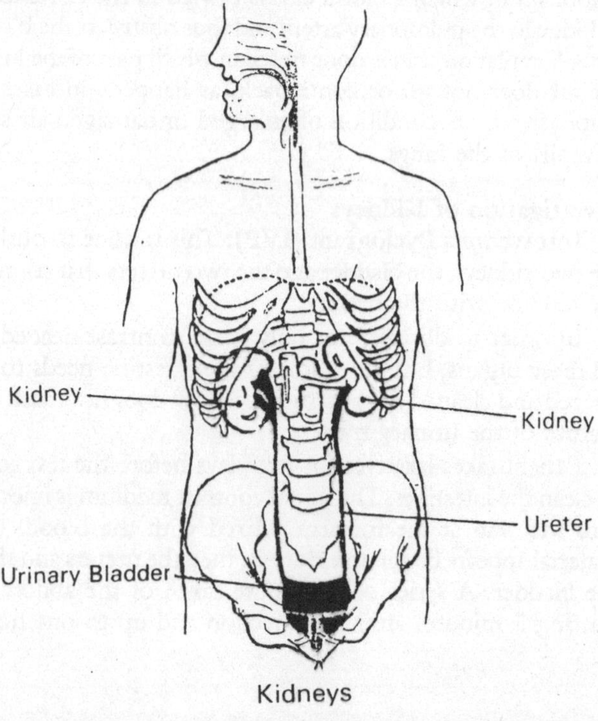

Kidneys

Investigation of Nervous System

Lumber Puncture and Myelogram: Under local anaesthetic a needle is inserted between 3rd and 4th lumber vertebra of the spine, so as to pierce the membranes over the spinal cord and reach the space where cerebro-spinal fluid (CSF) is situated. A small quantity of CSF is taken for bacteriological and chemical examination. Then a contrast medium is injected into the space, and patient screened on the X-ray table in straight and different tilted positions. Any narrowing or obstruction present in the spinal column is visualized on the X-ray screen and X-ray film taken wherever indicated.

As an after-effect, some headache may be noticed by the patient, which is relieved on resting.

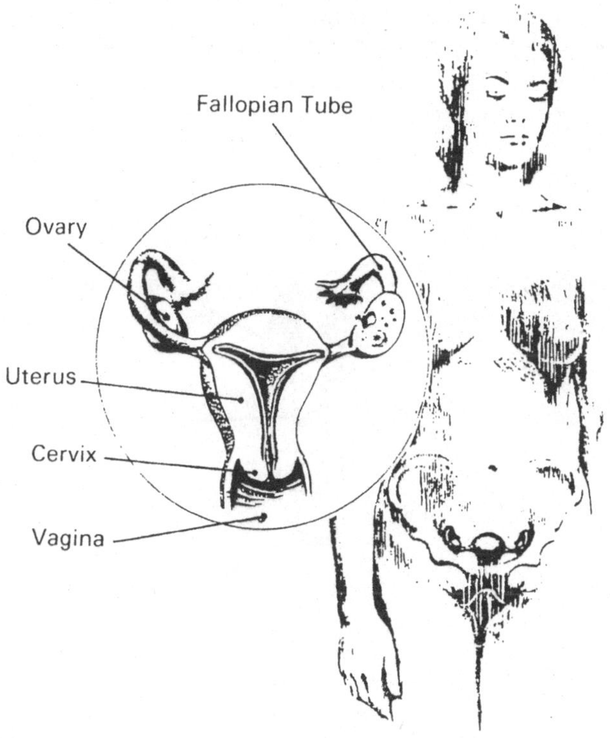

Female Genital Tract

Ultrasound and CT Scan: Both these procedures help in showing the site and extent of the lesion in a cancer patient.

Investigation of the Cervix of the Uterus

PAP Smear Test: This is performed routinely in all the women patients who come to the gynaecologist for some complaint. The walls of the vagina are held apart with a spatula so that the cervix is visible. A clean wooden spatula is smeared with the secretion on the surface of the cervix. This secretion is then smeared on a glass slide, fixed, stained and looked for evidence of cancer.

Biopsy of the Cervix: Biopsy of the cervix at the suspected site is taken and its histological examination reveals the diagnosis.

Investigation of the Thyroid

Thyroid Scan: The patient is given an iodine isotope in a drink to take. This isotope gets concentrated in the thyroid. Scanning and recording is done from there.

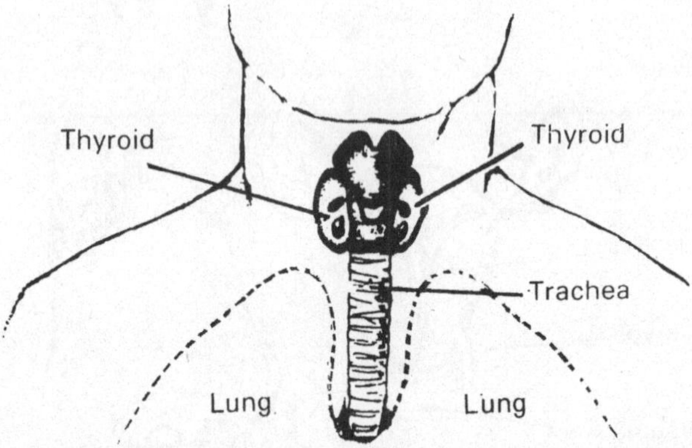

Thyroid Gland

This scan tells whether the whole or a part of the thyroid is hyper-or-hypo-functioning. Hyper-functioning or overactive thyroid is indicative of hyperthyroidism or Graves' disease, i.e. of excessive amount of the thyroid hormones in the bloodstream and hypo-functioning or underactive thyroid of diminution of these hormones. If a particular spot in a palpable nodule does not show any activity, it creates a suspicion of cancer.

Fine Needle Aspiration Biopsy: A needle is introduced into the suspected area of the thyroid and by means of a syringe fixed on the needle, the substance of the thyroid is sucked into the syringe. This may be fluid in case of a cyst, or have cells in it, which when examined histologically, give the diagnosis of the disease.

Investigation of a Lymph Node

Biopsy Examination: Lymph nodes or glands may be present on the surface of the body, for example, in the neck, axilla—the armpit or groin. From these places, it is not difficult to take out a whole gland and examine it histologically and also by culture for bacteria such as tubercle bocilli. But if the enlarged glands are present inside the body such as in the thorax or abdomen, then the part has to be operated upon and the gland removed.

Sometimes instead of removing the whole of the enlarged gland, a fine needle can be inserted in it and some part of it, the cells, sucked out with the syringe and examined histologically, which can reveal the diagnosis. The result can be available, depending upon the need, sometimes within an hour or a day or so.

Lymphangiogram: It is an X-ray of the lymph channels and the lymph glands of a particular part of the body, e.g. the legs or the abdomen. This is done to visualize the course, the dimensions of the vessels and the extent of the lymph glands.

The test is done in two parts spread over two days. A greenish-blue dye is first injected in the skin betweeen the first and second toes of each foot. The dye soon appears in fine lymph vessels on the skin over the feet.

Then with a very fine needle, a radio-opaque contrast dye is very slowly injected into one of the larger visible lymph vessels. This is a slow process and may take up to two to four hours. X-ray films are taken in between to see the extent of penetration of the dye in the legs and abdomen.

The next day, a further series of X-ray are done of the abdomen. In between and after the test, the patient will feel discomfort over the feet and legs, but it passess off soon.

Investigation of the Bones

Bone marrow Biopsy: Marrow is reached after piercing the bone. In some situations, for example, in children, at the upper end of the hip bone, the marrow can be reached easily, or in the case of adults at the sternum, front bone of the chest. Bone marrow is usually taken from the flat bones as they can be easily pierced compared to the long bones, which are thick and harder.

After infiltrating an anaesthetic fluid in the skin and deeper down, a thick-bored needle is inserted by a rotatory motion from the bone into the marrow. It does not give so much a pain as it does give little discomfort.

This examination provides a clear diagnosis in cases of leukaemia and other bone cancers.

5

Methods of Treatment

Cancer can be treated by any or all the following methods depending upon the site and the stage of the disease.

1. Surgical removal
2. Radiation therapy
3. Chemotherapy
4. Hormonal therapy

Which method should be used in a particular case, depends essentially on:

1. The type of cancer, and
2. The stage of the disease when diagnosed

It is necessary to see and recognise the cancer cell before a decision can be taken about the method of treatment. Some cancer cells respond to radiation, others don't; some cancer cells respond to one drug, others to another; many cancer cells respond better to a combination of drugs.

The stage of the disease at which a patient presents himself to the doctor, is very important in deciding the line of treatment. This is because survival rates are better for cancers that are localised or at primary stage than for those which have spread or at secondary stage.

The internationally recognised staging system is known as the TNM classification in which T defines the extent of the primary (t)umour, N defines the extent of the regional lymph (n)ode involvement, and M defines the presence or absence of (m)etastases.

The patient's history and physical examination provide a starting-point for planning treatment. It is usually necessary to perform specialized investigations to determine the type of cancer and extent of its dissemination or spread prior to selecting the treatment process.

Surgery

Surgery is usually indicated in cases of localized cancers. It may be done either alone or in combination with other lines of treatment such as radiation and chemotherapy.

If the cancer has not infiltrated into the surrounding areas and has not spread from the original site to different areas, then surgery may be all that is necessary. All the cancerous tissue has to be removed. In the process, even if a doubtful normal adjacent part is to be excised or surgically removed, this is done for the sake of safety and to prevent the recurrence of the cancer. The lymph glands enlarged or even suspicious, draining the area of cancer, are also resected or surgically removed.

Surgery is also resorted to in cases where the cancer is inoperable because of spread. This is done in order to remove any obstruction in a vital part of the body such as the intestines or bronchi of the lungs.

Surgery is also undertaken sometimes so that the patient is saved from very severe pain.

Radiation

Radiation involves the exposure of a selected area of the body to a source of ionising radiation or X-rays under carefully controlled conditions. Treatment planning involves accurate localization of the cancer and calculation of the total radiation dose to be given and dividing the same into daily fractions over a period of some days or weeks so that there is optimum response and minimum side-effects.

The calculation is done by the radiation therapist by taking care of all the facts of the case, including how sensitive to radiation are the cancer cells of a particular patient as diagnosed by a pathologist from a biopsy specimen. The measurement of the radiation given is counted in units called rads (radiation absorbed dose), i.e. the radiation absorbed by the tissues.

Small fractions of radiation given in divided doses over a period of many days or weeks, do less harm to the normal cells.

Radiation damages cells by interaction with DNA present in the nucleus of the cells thus preventing the normal reproduction of that cell. Fast-dividing cancer cells are more susceptible to being killed than the normal cells. The normal cells are also damaged in the process to some extent.

Side-effects of Radiation Treatment

A feeling of fatigue and diminished appetite are the commonest side effects, though not observed in all the patients.

Redness of the skin exposed to X-rays is not uncommon. When radiation is given over the abdomen, the patient may develop some amount of diarrhoea.

Radiation in the region of head and neck, may cause difficulty in swallowing.

Radiation effects on the bone marrow may occur if larger areas are treated. Minor decreases in lymphocyte count are common, but a frequent check on the peripheral blood is made throughout the treatment to adjust this if significant marrow suppression occurs.

Maintenance of adequate haemoglobin is important to the outcome of therapy since less oxygen in the blood (hypoxia) may render the cancer mass less sensitive to radiation damage.

Chemotherapy

Chemotherapy is the prevention or treatment of disease by the use of chemical substances. The term is sometimes restricted to the treatment of infectious diseases with antibiotics and other drugs or to the control of cancer with antimetabolites (that prevent cell growth) and similar drugs.

During the Second World War, research into the various aspects of the action of mustard gas which is ordinarily poisonous showed that this along with sulphur could destroy dividing cells in lymph nodes and the bone marrow. This harmful effect was harnessed to man's use for treating some lymphomas with nitrogen mustard. Thus was discovered the first cytotoxic drug against cancer, which damages or destroys cancer cells by inhibiting cell division.

Thereafter many naturally occurring substances were tested for anti-cancer activity on experimental animals resulting in the present availability of some 30 effective anti-cancer drugs.

Anti-cancer drugs are the treatment of choice for many widely disseminated cancers and serve as adjuncts to surgery and radiation in the treatment of localised ones.

The success of the various combinations of chemotherapy agents used in the treatment of some cancers, has brought hope to the patients.

Unfortunately, these drugs also affect normal cells particularly in bone marrow, skin, stomach lining, and foetal tissue and damage or destroy them, to some extent, resulting in many side-effects which are fairly serious. That is why the search for ideal anti-cancer drugs continues.

Categories of Anti-cancer Drugs

Various anti-cancer drugs developed over a period of three decades, can be grouped into different categories depending upon what function of the cancerous cells they disturb so as to kill them.

Alkylating Agents: They react chemically with DNA, the genetic material of the cell, which controls its division and function. Examples are, Busulphan, Chlorambucil, Cyclophosphamide.

Antimetabolites: They interfere with DNA production. Examples are, 5-Fluro-uracil, Methotrexate, 6-Mercaptopurine, Cytocine arbinoside.

Mitotic Inhibitor: They are plant alkaloids. They interfere directly with cell division. Examples are, Vincristine, Vinblastine, Vindesine.

Antibiotics: They are derived from different strains of bacteria. They can kill cancer cells. Examples are, Adriamycin, Actinomycin-D, Bleomycin, Mitomycin C.

Miscellaneous: These are drugs that work on cancer cells in ways different from the above categories. Examples are, Asparaginase, Hexamethylmelamine, Hydroxyurea.

Choice of Drug or Drug Combination

Some anti-cancer drugs are adequate in themselves to treat a particular cancer, but most of them are not. Since various drugs act differently, it was considered that a combination of them, each acting differently, would have a synergistic or increased effect. Dramatic results were produced by treating lymphomas or tumour of lymph node in this way. The four drug combination of Nitrogen mustard, Vincristine, Procarbazine and Prednisolone yielded complete remission in more than 80 per cent of patients with advanced Hodgkin's disease, whereas these same drugs used singly rarely produced remissions or lessening of symptoms in 15 to 20 per cent of cases. Similarly, combination chemotherapy for acute leukaemia or blood cancer increased the remission rates from 20 to 90 per cent.

Not only are different anti-cancer drugs used in combination to achieve better results, they are also used along with surgery and radiation.

Over the past 20 years, it has been shown that combination chemotherapy is valuable in many other cancers including cancer of the breast, ovary, lungs, testes and several of the childhood cancers.

With the development of combination chemotherapy, it became clear that the clinical course of different types of cancers could be influenced by cytotoxic drugs with cure in some and useful palliation—, i.e. which gives temporary relief from the symptoms—in many others.

It is possible to rank many kinds of cancers into different groups comprising those, for which chemotherapy contributes to cure, those for which effective control prolongs precious life, and those for which benefit is less certain or unproven.

Side-effects of Chemotherapy

Side-effects vary from drug to drug. But there are some which are more commonly seen and these are as follows:

Weakness: This is one of the commonest side-effects with most of the anti-cancer drugs. If the patient shows improvement in cancer situation after treatment, this side-effect may be felt less and less as the treatment goes on.

Decreased Appetite: Decreased appetite or even loss of appetite may be observed for some days after the administration of the drug. The appetite may improve gradually.

Nausea and Vomiting: This is observed with most of the drugs. In some cases it may be so severe, as to make the doctor reconsider his decision to change to an other drug. Mild to moderate symptoms can be contiolled with anti-emetic drugs.

Sore Mouth: The lining cells of the mucous membrane in the mouth get damaged with chemotherapeutic agents and so there is sore mouth and difficulty in eating. Liquid diet taken with a straw proves helpful to the patient.

Diarrhoea: All along the lining of the intestinal tract, as with the mucous membrane in the mouth, there is damage and inflammation. That is why the food passes by quickly without being absorbed properly, leading on to diarrhoea. Easily digestible diet and drugs that can lead to formation of proper stools, help the patient.

Hair Loss: Many of the anti-cancer drugs cause loss of hair. This is because the hair cells divide rapidly (like those present in the mucous membrane of the intestine) and hence are more susceptible to the action of these drugs. This hair loss is a temporary process and after some time the hair re-grow as before.

Response of Different Cancers to Chemotherapy

Leads to Cure	Leads to Prolongation of Life	Marginal Benefit	No Benefit
Blood cancer or acute lymphoblastic leukaemia in children	Cancer of the breast	Cancer of the stomach	Cancer of the lung, squamous cell type
Cancer of lymphatic system or Burkitt's lymphoma	Cancer of the ovaries	Cancer of the pancreas	Cancer of the colon
Hodgkin's disease—a malignant tumour of lymphatic system	Cancer of the lung, small-cell anaplastic type	Bone cancer or Myeloma	Cancer of the oesophagus
Wilms' tumour or tumour of the kidney common among children	Non-Hodgkin's lymphoma	Soft tissues arcoma	Cancer of the skin or Melanoma
Cancer of the muscle or Rhabdomyosarcoma	Chronic lymphocytic leukaemia	Cancer of the urinary bladder	
Cancer of the testes or Teratoma of the testes	Acute myeloid leukaemia	Cancer of the thyroid	
Cancer of the placenta or Choriocarcinoma	Brain cancer or Medulloblastoma		
Cancer of bone common among children or Ewing's sarcoma			

Skin Rashes: Itchy rashes, red and raised above the surface of the skin are not uncommon with some drugs. They disturb the sleep of the patient and are generally very annoying. Soothing skin lotions provide some help.

Bone Marrow Suppression: The cells in the bone marrow are fast dividing ones—faster dividing than those of the intestinal lining or of the hair root. Anti-cancer drugs when they act on the fast dividing cancer cells, also act more or less similarly on the dividing bone marrow cells, killing them in the process. The result is that the RBC, WBC and platelets which are formed in the bone marrow, have their rate of formation much diminished, and so less of them come into the bloodstream. The result is anaemia due to less of RBC, granulocytopenia and subsequent danger of infection, and thrombocytopenia and bleeding from various sources. Utmost care is needed to prevent suppression of bone marrow, or to replace by blood transfusion the loss of blood cells.

Loss of Reproductive Function: In mâles, anti-cancer drugs diminish the number of spermatozoa being released from the testes, and in females they cause stoppage of menstrual cycles (amenorrhoea) leading on to infertility.

This infertility may not be permanent, and reproductive power may get restored after the stoppage of the drug.

Chemotherapy is not given during pregnancy as it may lead to termination of pregnancy or malformation of the foetus.

Hormonal Treatment of Certain Cancers

Cancers which develop in organs that are known to be under hormonal control, sometimes retain hormonal dependency. Withdrawing the source of the hormone in some such cases, lessens the growth of cancer. Cancers of the breast, prostate, uterus and thyroid are the ones amenable to hormonal treatment.

Previously, the adrenal glands or the pituitary gland were removed surgically for this purpose. But now the same effect is produced by medical rather than surgical means. Cancer response to Tamoxifen and Aminoglutethamide may take 6 to 12 weeks to manifest. Hence, it is necessary to wait for this period before making decisions about further management.

Androgen, the male sex hormone, may produces response in about 20 per cent of patients with breast cancer, particularly in post-menopausal women with bone metastasis. Oestrogen the female sex hormone is useful in the palliation of prostate cancer.

Some cancers of the thyroid remain under the influence of thyroid-stimulating hormone (TSH) and the administration of thyroid hormones may be useful as a result of its inhibiting pituitary secretion of TSH.

The major advantage of hormonal therapy over chemotherapy is that the side-effects are usually less severe than those associated with cytotoxic drugs. Tamoxifen rarely causes toxicity but aminoglutethamide can cause drowsiness, depression and transient skin rashes in some patients. The use of oestrogen in elderly men with prostate cancer warrants special caution in view of its known propensity to aggravate the fluid retention that may be harmful to the patients also suffering from a heart disease.

6

Common Symptoms & Their Treatment

Cancer can cause many symptoms. These symptoms may be categorised as under:

1. Common to any cancer,
2. Others that depend upon the site of cancer, and
3. The type of cancer. Some symptoms are caused by the treatment by means of chemotherapy and radiation.

Loss of Appetite and Weight

Loss of appetite and weight are the commonest symptoms of cancer. These may be due to:

1. Poor appetite, so that there is less intake of food.
2. Cancer tissue burns excessive energy of the body.
3. Vomiting and diarrhoea allow less food to be absorbed.

In order to increase the appetite more appetising food may be given. Appetizers like mild alcoholic drinks may be considered. Sometimes steroids prove helpful, where other measures have failed.

Nausea and Vomiting

These are common symptoms after chemotherapy or

radiation. When severe, they may be difficult to tolerate even by a well-informed patient.

Anti-vomiting (anti-emetic) tablets are suggested for mild or moderate cases. These include Largactil tablets (Chlorpromazine) Stemetil (Prochlorperazine).

Diarrhoea

This is more often the effect of the chemotherapy treatment, but sometimes may be due to cancer itself. Anti-diarrhoeal drugs like Codeine Phosphate 1 to 2 tablets three times daily, and Lomotil, two tablets three times a day, are helpful.

Constipation

This may be due to diminished appetite or loss of appetite, inactivity, change in diet, or even due to pain-relieving drugs.

Stool softeners such as liquid Paraffin, are helpful.

Lack of Sleep (Insomnia)

Many of the symptoms of cancer or the depression and anxiety associated with it, can make the patient lose sleep. Appropriate treatment of the symptoms, may provide the patient, the much needed relief. Sedatives and hypnotics like Diazepam can be helpful. Depression can be helped by tricyclic drugs like Depsol, Depsonil.

Pain

Pain is not an invariable symptom associated with cancer. As many as half the cancers in even an advanced stage, do not cause pain. But where it is present, it may be continuous and gradually increase in intensity and may be difficult to bear.

A pain-relieving drug is needed to be taken regularly so that the pain is kept at bay. The choice of the drug depends upon the severity of the pain. This topic is discussed in detail in a subsequent chapter.

Shortness of Breath

Shortness of breath, often with cough, is not uncommon in advanced cancer. The commonest causes are:

Cancer in the lung.

Collection of fluid in the pleural cavity around the lung.

Scarring and fibrosis of the lungs.

Infection in the lung, such as pneumonia in a case of lung cancer.

Treatment depends upon the cause. Cancer will need either surgery, radiation or chemotherapy.

Cough

It is treated after finding out the cause. Cough caused by infection in a case of lung cancer is treated by giving appropriate antibiotic. Irritant cough without much phlegm is suppressed by a cough mixture containing Codeine or related compounds.

Urinary Incontinence

This distressing symptom is caused by a variety of causes. Urinary infections cause increased frequency and occasionally incontinence. Approprate antibiotic is indicated.

Cancer in the pelvis, irritating or pressing on the bladder can cause increased frequency or incontinence. Radiation and/or chemotherapy may help.

If continence continues, then a catheter is passed through the urethra which drains the bladder into a container, without soiling the patient's bed. Care is necessary to see that no infection enters the urethra and the urinary bladder.

Obstruction in the Bowel

Obstruction or blockage of the bowel is most often caused by cancer of the large bowel. It usually starts slowly with occasional attack just like colic pain in the abdomen. The pain is often accompanied by loud bowel sounds and swelling of the abdomen.

The symptoms of complete bowel obstruction are:

Colicky abdominal pain

Nausea

Vomiting

Constipation may become so complete that even wind is not passed.

The following measures are suggested as part of the treatment:

No food or drinks are taken by mouth.
Fluids are given intraveneously.
In case of severe vomiting, a tube is passed through the nose into the patient's stomach and excess fluids sucked out.

In some cases, the obstruction settles down with this treatment. If it does not, then surgical operation is performed.

Collection of Fluid in the Abdomen (Ascites)

Sometimes cancer in the abdomen causes fluid to accumulate and this can lead to uncomfortable swelling and also difficulty in breathing.

A wide-bored needle or a plastic catheter is passed through the skin of the abdomen and fluid is drawn up into a syringe.

Sore Mouth

This may be due to drug reaction, vitamin deficiency, aphthous or small ulcers, fungal infections or bacterial infections.

Careful cleansing of the mouth is very important. For fungal infections, anti-fungal lozenges are helpful. Miconazole (Daktarin gel) is used to rinse the mouth at least four times a day. Ketoconazole is also used.

For anti-cancer drugs producing sores in the mouth, the treatment is to keep the mouth hygienically clean.

Difficulty in Swallowing

Cancer in or near the oesophagus, i.e. the food pipe can cause difficulty in swallowing (dysphagia). Some cancers respond to treatment and pressure upon the oesophagus may be removed, but many of them don't. In such a case, an operation is performed to insert a tube from the upper end through the cancer to the lower end.

7

Management of Cancer Related Problems

Various problems arise in cancer patients during their illness. These may be related to the treatment which the patient undergoes. These problems need effective management.

Management of Pain

Whenever a patient with cancer complains of pain, a careful diagnostic work up is required. Such a work up is designed to define as precisely as possible, the cause of pain. When a cancer causes pain, it does so by different mechanisms. These are:

1. Compression of nervous tissue, i.e. peripheral nerve root, or spinal cord, by cancer infiltration directly, or by bone in the case of pathologic bone fracture or vertebral collapse.
2. Direct infiltration of nervous tissue or interference with its blood supply by the cancer mass.
3. Obstruction of a passage, e.g. bowel.
4. Inflammation in pain-sensitive structures directly or by infection.
5. Cancer-associated nerve sense disturbance (neuropathy) caused probably by some secretion from the cancer cells.

Once the cause of pain is established, it is managed either by removal of the cause or by suppression of pain.

Removal of the Cause

Surgery: Removal of an obstructing colon cancer.

Radiation therapy: Directed to painful bone metastases or to the whole liver beset with painful metastases.

Chemotherapy: Combination chemotherapy in breast cancer metastatic to bone.

Miscellaneous: Antibiotics for an infected skin ulcer, corticosteroids for cerebral oedema and its attendant headache in primary and metastatic brain cancers.

Suppression of Pain

When a direct attack on the cause of pain is not possible, or when the response to primary pain control is delayed, symptomatic approach is indicated. Here treatment is directed at modification of neural processing of the painful stimulus or of its perception. Diverse and often complementary therapeutic measures are available ranging from the administration of Aspirin to major neurosurgical operation.

For many patients, especially those with chronic pain and short life expectancies, pain management is centred around the use of analgesics. Mild analgesics like Aspirin or Patacetamal, provide satisfactory relief for a while. The use of stronger analgesic drugs (including potent narcotics) then becomes necessary.

Anti-anxiety and anti-depression medication may also be needed in the control of pain in many cases of cancer.

Management of Infections

Infection is the most serious complication in cases of acute leukaemia. Infection in general, accounts for approximately 70 per cent of the symptoms and as subsequent cause of death in patients with acute leukaemias.

Substantial advances have been made over the last decade in the prevention and treatment of infection in cancer patients. Different types of infection occur as a result of abnormalities in post-defense mechanisms. Patients with diminished leukocytes in the blood (granulocytopaenia), are likely to develop infection with gram-negative bacilli such as S. Aureus.

Role of Antibiotics

Treatment with broad spectrum antibiotics, is usually helpful. Susceptibility of the infecting organism to the antibiotics and subsequent increase in leukocyte counts, are indicators of good prognosis.

Role of Blood Transfusion

The newer, more effective anti-cancer drug regimens that have evolved for the treatment of both leukaemia and other cancers cause substantial bone marrow suppression.

The use of these treatment regimens, many a time, needs whole blood or granulocyte transfusion as a supportive measure. This has proved very helpful in the treatment of acute leukaemias with significantly better results. Prophylactic white blood cell (granulocyte) transfusions can even prevent serious infection in granulocytopenic patients. Numerous reports have described groups of patients with serious infection not improving on antibiotic therapy, which have resolved with the addition of granulocytic transfusions.

Granulocyte transfusion is also indicated if the patient has a severe infection not responding to appropriate antibiotics, and there is likelihood of prolonged periods of granulocytopenia.

Fungal infections are increasingly recognised as pathogens, particularly in patients treated for substantial periods with broad-spectrum anti-bacterial antibiotics. Prompt therapy with Amphotericin-B has been shown to be efficacious even during continuing graulocytopenia.

Cancer patients are liable to develop a deficiency of immune response so that they are more susceptible to infections than patients suffering from other diseases. This aspect has to be kept in mind and wherever necessary and possible, this deficiency is repaired. Control of cancer, by itself restores the immune deficiency.

Infection prevention is a critical issue and a major responsibility of those who care for cancer patients. Bolstering of host defense mechanisms, avoidance of unnecessary invasive or traumatic procedures, suppression of organisms colonizing at or near common sites of infection, and reduction of acquisition of hospital-associated organisms, contribute to reduction of the incidence of infection.

Management of Problems Related to Surgery

Surgery performed on gastro-intestinal and urinary tracts creates its own problems of getting rid of the faces or the urine which now cannot be evacuated through normal openings. New openings may be/can be made by the following

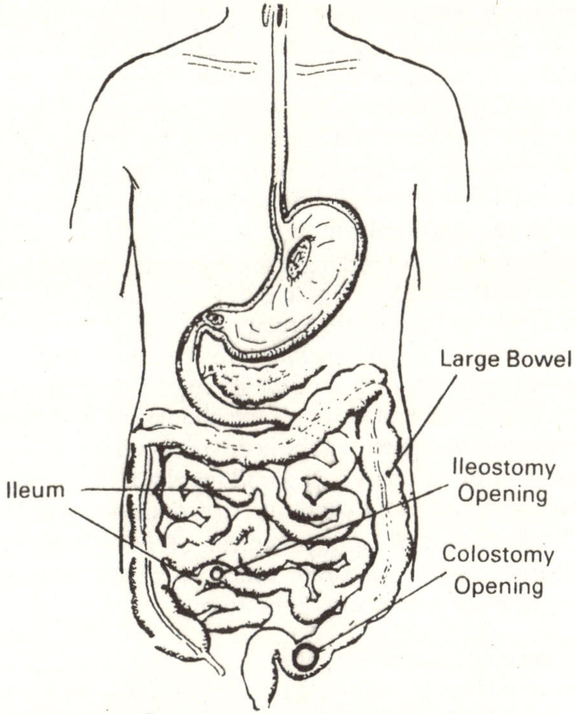

Colostomy Opening and Ileostomy Opening at the Sigmoid Region of the Large Bowel

operations. These new openings made need constant and effective care.

Colostomy: When the opening is formed from the colon, the stoma is called a colostomy. Stoma may be made from any part of the colon, depending upon where the disease is. When the opening is formed from the ileum part of the small bowel, the stoma is known as an ileostomy. This ostomy is made using the ileum, the part of the small intestine that is farthest from the stomach and nearest to the colon. This is done where the colon and the rectum is removed.

As there is no longer a colon to absorb water and form solid stools, the ileostomy discharges liquid which flows almost continuously. This contains digestive enzymes, so the ileostomy stoma is made to protrude up to an inch into the appliance so that the skin is protected. This is important because the enzymes may digest the skin.

Urostomy: In the cancer of the bladder, it may be necessary to totally remove the bladder. This surgical removal of bladder is called urostomy. The ureters, the tubes that connect the kidneys and bladder, may be brought directly up to the skin, or may be connected to the ileum (part of the small bowel) which is brought up to the skin as a stoma. This is called an ileal conduit.

The operation of making ileal conduit, is so called because the surgeon converts a segment of the ileum (about 15 cm) into a pipe, or conduit for urinary drainage. The ureters are disconnected from the bladder (which is usually removed) and are joined to one end of the ileum, the other end of the ileum being brought through the abdominal wall to form the stoma. The segment of the ileum removed from the small intestine survives on its own blood supply and the rest of the bowel is rejoined and continues to work normally.

There is no voluntary control of the stoma which discharges a drop of urine every 10 to 20 seconds. A urostomy bag is worn over the stoma.

Management After Surgery

After an ostomy operation, the patient loses voluntary control over the discharge of the wastes concerned, and he has to wear a special appliance for the collection of this waste. With care and training, the patient learns very soon how to manage it and thus lives a perfectly normal life.

The excreta coming out of the intestinal ostomy is different in colour from that one is used to seeing. The effects of various foods and medications are apparent in the excreta. It smells more than the ordinary stool, as unformed stool has more odour. The texture is different and also the volume is more, because it is more of liquid than dry. The noisy stoma that sounds like the grumbling of a hungry stomach is unusual from the normal sounds and may be embarrassing to a new patient.

The patient and his relatives must be informed on all these aspects before the operation, so that they know and are prepared for it.

Immediately after the operation, all care should be extended to the patient by the hospital staff and the relatives. He should learn to do all the management himself so that he develops confidence in himself.

Management of Nutrition

Wasting (Cachexia)

Cancer frequently leads to widely recognized but poorly understood syndrome known as cachexia. The manifestations of this syndrome are weakness, loss of weight and appetite (anorexia). The patient appears ill and emaciated. The cause of anorexia remains complex and unclear. Muscle biopsies from breast and colon cancer patients show fat content of the muscles to be half of non-cancer patients. There is also an increased break down of proteins in the muscles.

There has been an increasing awareness of cachexia in patients with cancer. In one autopsy series, more than 22 per cent of the patients died without identifiable cause other than cancer cachexia. These patients did not die of their cancer, but of the systemic effects of their cancer that produced the debilitating syndrome that is cachexia. In addition to contributing to mortality, the malnutrition and wasting present serious symptomatic problems.

Cause of Wasting (Cachexia): The cause is not well understood, but there are some contributing factors.

1. Cancers at specific sites like oesophagus produce mechanical obstruction to passage of food.
2. It has been postulated that metabolic demands are increased in cancer patients due to competition by cancer cells for nutrition. Various studies have demonstrated increased nutrients consumption in large sarcomas.
3. Other mechanisms like abnormalities of smell and taste, deranged nervous system control and presence of cancer cell secretions in the blood, are all implicated.
4. Besides the cancer, treatment can also influence nutritional status of the patient. Chemotherapy and radiation therapy can lead to malnutrition by causing mucositis, enteritis and vomiting, while the stress of surgery produces a hyper-catabolic state. Nutritional consequences of cancer chemotherapy are secondary to its side-effects such as nausea, vomiting, oral pain, diarrhoea and fever.

Management: Adequate nutritional support is necessary. When voluntary oral intake is unsatisfactory and the gastro-intestional tract is functional, feeding via gastric tube is indicated.

When gastrointestinal tract cannot be used for nutritional support, total intravenous nutrition is essential, until tube or oral feeding can be resorted to.

It is likely that by offering such nutritional support before, during and after the treatment, clinical response may improve and also tolerance to therapy.

Total intravenous nutrition is a newer and effective method of nutritional support through which carbohydrates and fats for calories and amino acids for nitrogen requirements, are given. It is useful before the treatment as well as after the treatment with radiation and chemotherapy. However, this involves close monitoring of metabolic needs and careful adjustment of mineral and trace metals in the body.

Management of Dental Problems

Patients with undiagnosed leukaemias may first seek care from the dentist. In these individuals, oral symptoms are among the earliest common complaints. There is a direct relationship between low platelet counts and increased episodes of serious bleeding from the gum in these patients; platelet tansfusions proved effective in checking bleeding. It was also noticed that fever and septicaemia predisposed to serious bleeding with rapid utilization of platelets and poor survival of transfused platelets. Thus, more frequent transfusions are needed in such clinical situations, also as prophylaxis.

The oral changes start with a reddening of the inside of the mouth observed at the end of the first week of treatment. By the middle of the second week, white patches appear on the lining (mucosa) of the lips, cheeks and tongue. The irritation becomes progressively more severe week by week. A sloughing of the mucosa occurs by the third week, and by the 4th and 5th week, the lips and corners of the mouth have an ulcerated appearance. The mucosa may become very painful, the discomfort being so severe that the patient resists chewing and swallowing.

Alkaline mouthwash to which a large spoonful of milk of magnesia is added, gives some relief. Rinsing of the mouth with topical xylocaine before meals, may help the patient to eat. Another effect of radiation therapy is the severe depression of salivary secretion, leading to marked, persistent and irreversible sensation of dryness of the mouth. The dosage required to produce it, has been reported as 1500 rads to 2000 rads. The time required to produce the condition has been reported as early as at 2 to 6 hours after radiation to up to 3 weeks.

Management of Terminal Phase

A difficult part of the management of cancer patient is when he enters the terminal phase of his illness. When it becomes apparent that active measures to arrest further growth of the cancer are no longer proving effective, it is more important than ever to provide support and attention to the alleviation of distressing symptoms.

Psychological support is the most important aspect. But this has to be supplemented with positive measures to relieve pain, to ensure adequate and appropriate nutrition and treat specific symptoms such as cough, nausea, vomiting, pain, etc.

An individual patient's reaction to the inevitability of death from a fatal disease depends on a host of interrelated variables including his or her cultural and religious background, age, education, the duration of the illness, reaction of dependents, etc. A period of initial disbelief and denial is often replaced by resentment and anger. This, in turn, is followed by a period of depression, which is almost universal. Many patients, with or without medical intervention, enter a final phase of peacefully accepting the inevitability of death.

When to tell patients that they have a terminal illness, is a matter of experience and judgment that cannot be easily mastered. Avoiding such discussions can only enhance the patients sense of loneliness and isolation.

It is not always appropriate to present all of the facts to a patient, especially on a single occasion, and time must be spent to determine the patient's awareness of his situation. Non-committal, even ambiguous statements about the future may be appropriate but the patient should never be told what is known to be untrue.

The most important principle of managing terminal illness is to provide adequate time for talking with the patient. The doctor must learn to develop the ability to listen to the patient and to learn from him how best to provide him psychological support.

Help of an appropriate religious person or social worker is very useful in such a situation.

8

Prevention of Cancer

Prevention of cancer attempts to eliminate the disease by protecting the individual and the community from the causative agent. This is called primary prevention. This involves environmental monitoring of cancer-causing agents (carcinogens), identification of high risk groups and procedures to abolish any contact between the carcinogen and the host.

Prevention also aims at correcting those pathological states which have already been produced, and which if allowed to continue, may end in cancer. This is called secondary prevention. The identification and management of such cases made possible through mass screening techniques applicable to cancer of the cervix, lung, mouth, stomach and liver, fall into this category.

The types of cancer prevailing in India are predominantly such as can be prevented and/or detected early by simple techniques and methods available today.

Primary Prevention

The most important point under primary prevention of cancer is imparting proper education to people about factors that can lead to cancer. This knowledge is woefully lacking in our country even amongst the educated people, leave aside the village folks. The writing of this book is a step in this direction.

The aim of imparting this education is to make people aware of the dangers that they run when they expose themselves to cancer-causing agents.

The following are some of the clearly preventable cancers.

Oral Cancer

Oral cancer is a typically preventable, detectable and treatable cancer and yet one of the most prevalent in India.

That tobacco and its products can give rise to cancer inside the mouth was first pointed out in 1915. The doctor who made such an observation wrote: "The worst cancer of the tongue I have recently seen was in a woman. All the left half of the tongue and the half of the right, was cancerous. I asked her how it began and she said: 'I have all my life, taken a small tooth brush in my right hand, dipped it in snuff (containing tobacco powder) and rubbed it hard on my tongue on the left."

The incidence of mouth cancer is the highest in India, mainly because of the widely-prevalent habit of chewing tobacco. Mouth cancer forms one-third of all the cancer cases in India. In other countries, its incidence is much less: USSR 4.6 per cent, UK 4.27 per cent, USA 3.4 per cent, Japan 2.6 per cent, Scandinavian countries 2.5 per cent.

Those who are in the habit of chewing tobacco daily, run eight times more risk of developing mouth cancer than do the non-chewers. The risk is higher when chewing tobacco is started at an earlier age. A definite dose-effect relationship has also been observed. How long the quid is kept in the mouth is also relevant. It has been observed that some of the tobacco chewers keep tobacco in the mouth while they go to sleep; this increases greatly the risk of getting cancer. The risk increases further if the quid is kept only on one side.

If tobacco chewing can be controlled, there would be a substantial reduction of cancer.

Lung Cancer

Cancer of the lung is most prevalent in males in Western countries and is also said to be increasing in India. It is known to be associated with smoking cigarettes. It is generally accepted that there is a causal connection between cigarette smoking and lung cancer. Epidemiological studies have shown that there is a clear relationship between the number of cigarette smoked and the incidence of lung cancer. Giving up smoking decreases the susceptibility to lung cancer, in proportion to the number of years that smoking has been given up.

The longer a cigarette is, the more tar and nicotine one inhales. The last half of the cigarette contains twice as much tar and nicotine as the first half. This applies to 'king-sized' cigarettes also.

Further, no method of treating tobacco or filtering the smoke has yet been demonstrated to be effective in materially reducing or eliminating the hazards of lung cancer.

So, smokers are advised to stop smoking or to drastically reduce it.

Uterine Cervix Cancer

Cancer of the uterine cervix is the most important cancer in terms of its frequency and also of its potential of control. Early marriage and multiple pregnancies are significant factors for the prevalence of this cancer. Avoidence of these, can be a safety measure against this cancer.

Cancer of Penis

Cancer of penis is almost unknown among the Jews in whom circumcision is done within one week of birth. It is rare among Muslims too in whom circumcision is done between the ages of four and fourteen years. But it is fairly common among the Hindus who do not practice circumcision. This is not to say that everyone should get circumcised, but the purpose can be served by keeping the skin over the penis hygienically clean.

General Measures

1. Improvement of personal hygiene such as of mouth, skin and genitals will help to reduce the incidence of certain types of cancer.

2. Control of air pollution can be regarded as another preventive measure.

3. All drugs, cosmetics, and food additives should be tested for carcinogenesis.

4. Special efforts should be made to reduce the amount of radiation (including medical radiation) received by each individual to a minimum without reducing the benefits.

5. Measures to protect workers from carcinogenic agents should be enforced in industries.

Use of pesticides of various types is being recognized as a source of many diseases, including cancers. Use of DDT/BHC, Malathion and such other pesticides should be reduced and regulated.

6. Legislation has also a role in primary prevention. The State has promulgated legislation with regard to air pollution, and for inserting statutory warning on cigarette packets. Legislation, however, needs to be enforced strictly.

7. Cancer registeration is an important means of prevention of cancer. It provides a base for assessing the magnitude of the problem in an area and country and for planning the necessary services. It provides opportunities to study:

Incidence and prevalence of cancer.

Geographic differences in cancer.

Clustering (in time, space or person) of specific cancers.

Effect of socio-economic variables upon cancer incidence.

Effect of occupational exposures upon cancer rates.

Influence of other environmental exposures upon the development of cancer.

Length of survival as related to specific cancer treatment.

8. Diet and human life-styles have a potential effect on cancer in a community. Cancer of the gastrointestinal tract are probably closely related to diet and life-styles. Food,

particularly fat, having even traces of pesticides in it, can prove carcinogenic in the long run.

Cancer is a multi-stage phenomenon. Interruption is possible at different stages.

You May Prevent Cancer if You ...
Avoid smoking, especially cigarettes. Avoid drinking excessive alcohol. Avoid excessive sun exposure, if you are light-skinned. Avoid using birth control pills indiscriminately. Avoid using oestrogens for menopausal symptoms except under specific guide-lines. Avoid early or frequent intercourse, especially with multiple sex partners. Try to have only two or three pregnancies, after the age of 20, but do not wait until after 30 to have your first.

For Prevention of Cancer
Avoid foods containing nitrites and nitrates, these are found mainly in preserved meats, e.g. bacon and other cured meats. Avoid colour additives as much as possible. This is often difficult as many foods contain them, and a sensible balance may have to be accepted. Wash insecticides off all fresh fruit and vegetables. Avoid artificial sweeteners if possible, e.g. saccharin.

Secondary Prevention

As already stated, it aims at correcting those pathological states which have already been produced, and which if allowed to continue, may lead to symptoms of cancer.

Screening for cancer comes under this category and the two important cancers that can come under this programme are:

1. Cancer of the uterine cervix.
2. Cancer of the breast.

Uterine Cervix Cancer

In many Western countries, deaths from cervical cancer have been reduced by up to 50 per cent in the past 20 years. During this time, there has been increasing awareness of the importance of early diagnosis and a concerted effort to screen for the disease using the cervical smear technique or pap test.

Cells from the cervix are examined under a microscope after they have been scraped from the lining of the cervix. Many of the cancers found by this method are localized to the surface and are called *in-situ* cancers. Cervical cancer, when caught at this stage, is nearly always curable (more than 95 per cent).

These tests should be done on women after the age of 40 years in symptomless cases, and in those who having abnormal vaginal bleeding or persistent vaginal discharge, even earlier. Women with abnormal cells that may represent a pre-cancer change (called dysplasia) will need to have a biopsy of the cervix.

An important and interesting study on the prevalence of cervical cancer and the role of certain environmental factors in its etiology in urban and rural population of the district of Agra was carried out from 1967 to 1970, at the Cancer Research Centre, Department of Pathology, S.N. Medical College, Agra by Dr. Usha K. Luthra. A 10 per cent sample of the total married female population of 20 years old and above, in the urban and rural areas of the Agra district was studied. The subjects were examined clinically, and cervical smears were taken. A total of 26,533 subjects were examined clinically and cytologically by the Pap test. It was found that the average annual crude prevalence rate was 210 per 100,000 women, showing that Agra was a high risk area for cervical cancers. The prevalence rate of cervical cancer in Muslims was 3.20 per 1000, being approximately half of the Hindu women, i.e. 6.62 per 1000. Women who were married at the age of 14 years and below, had more than three times the prevalence of cervical cancer than women who were married at 20 years of age and above. Prevalence rate of uterine cervical cancer being twice high in Hindu females as compared with the Muslim females, may be due to the cultural fact that Muslim males are circumcised while Hindu males are not circumcised.

Studies such as cited above, provide enough information about the prevalence of cancer in an area and the means to be employed to prevent it.

Breast Cancer

Breast cancer is one of the common cancers in women. The breast is easily examined by self or the doctor.

Self-examination of the breast is done after learning the technique from the specialist doctor. This should be done monthly. This is the first line of screening and a careful examination should pick up a small lump if present. Women still having their periods need to examine their breasts at the same time each month as the shape and feel of the breasts changes with the menstrual cycle. The best time to examine the breast is 7 days after the start of each period. Breast examination by a doctor is usually got done every 6 months.

Self-Examination of Breasts*

1. Look at your breasts in the mirror with your arms by your side, then with them up in the air. Look for puckering.

2. Lie down, and with the left arm behind the head, examine the left breast with the flat of the right hand fingers. Work from the upper, inner quarter and then towards the nipple.

3. Feel round the nipple, then continue to the lower inner quarter.

4. Put your arm by your side, then working from outside the breast area, feel towards the lower outer quarter, the

---

*For further reading consult *Breast Self-Examination* by Dr. Albert R. Milan, M.D., published by Orient Paperbacks, Delhi.

nipple, then the upper outer quarter.

5. Check the breast tissue across the top of the breast to the armpit.

6. Feel inside the armpit.

For the right breast begin with the upper inner quarter and your right arm behind your head.

There is an other specialised screening test for breast cancer called mammography. This is a special X-ray of the breast useful for detecting cancers too small to be felt. This is done in patients at high risk, usually after the age of 50 years.

All patients with a breast lump should be seen by a specialist so that it may be looked at closely and if necessary biopsied. The majority of breast lumps that are biopsied, do not contain cancer (they are benign), but this can only be proved by examining the lump under a microscope. The decision whether to perform a biopsy or not, can only be made by a specialist and general practitioners should refer all patients with a breast lump immediately to a breast clinic.

Warning Signs of Breast Cancer

Unusual difference in size or shape of the breasts.
Alterations in the position of either nipple.
Retraction (turning in) of either nipple.
Puckering (dimple) of the skin surface over the breast.
Unusual rash on the breast or nipple.
Unusual prominence of the veins over either breast.
Unusual discrete lump or nodule in any part of either breast on Palpation.

9

Leukaemias

These are commonly called 'blood cancer'. In fact, these are cancer of the bone marrow which produces the cells, viz. red and white blood cells and the platelets that circulate in the blood. In this condition, the white blood cells produced in the bone marrow are cancerous and immature. They are also produced in number much more than the normal cells. That is why the condition is called leukaemia, literally meaning white blood. The other cells produced in the marrow such as the red blood cells and the platelets are produced less.

Untreated, the leukaemias are progressive and fatal; death occurs from anaemia, bleeding (haemorrhage) or repeated infections. The course may vary from a few weeks to several years depending upon the severity of the condition and the type of white blood cells involved. Some leukaemias run an acute course, others a chronic one. The leukaemic process effects either the precursors of the lymphocytes, or the granulocytes also called myeloid cells.

Of all the varieties of leukaemia, acute lymphoblastic leukaemia (ALL) involving the precursors of lymphocyte, i.e. the lymphoblasts, is the commonest in children; it forms one-third of all childhood cancers. It occurs between the age of 2 to 7 years, and is uncommon after the age of 15 years.

In adults, the common acute leukaemia is non-lymphocytic (ANLL), also called acute myelogenous leukaemia (AML) because it involves myeloid cells.

Acute lymphoblastic leukaemia, the type commonly found in children, is rare in adults.

Leukaemias are thus classified as:

Acute lymphoblastic and acute non-lymphoblastic (also called acute myeloid).

Chronic lymphocytic and non-lymphocytic.

Causes of Leukaemias

In the majority of cases the cause of leukaemia is unknown. Several factors, however, are known to be associated with the development of leukaemia. These are:

1. **Ionising Radiation:** There was an undoubted increase in leukaemia incidence following the atomic bombing of the Japanese cities. A striking increase in leukaemia was also observed after the use of X-ray therapy to control an arthritic condition of the spine called ankylosing spondylitis.

2. **Cytotoxic Drugs:** These, particularly alkylating agents used in the treatment of cancer may induce leukaemia after a latent period of several years.

3. **Exposure to Benzene:** This is a chemical compound used in industries.

4. **Retrovirus:** It has been found to be associated with one type of leukaemia.

Acute Leukaemias

Symptoms

Tiredness.

Bleeding after slight injury.

Frequent infections.

Lump in the abdomen which is found out to be the spleen.

Discomfort or pain over the bones.

Loss of weight.

Diminished appetite.

The onset is after abrupt with flu-like symptoms and fatigue.

There may be fever, malaise and a rapidly progressive anaemia.

Bleeding from the nose (epistaxis), bleeding from the gums or bleeding patches in the skin called purpura, are common and are due largely to reduction in platelet count in the blood (thrombocytopenia). Sore throat and ulcers in the mouth or pharynx are frequent, due to reduction in normal polymorpho-nuclear leukocytes.

Diagnosis

Routine: Blood: RBC counts and Hb are low, TLC counts are high, and there are immature white cells in the blood.

ESR is raised.

Platelet counts are diminished.

Special: Bone marrow biopsy and histological examination of the same helps in establishing the diagnosis.

Additional: X-ray of the chest indicates if the lungs have been involved in the leukaemic process.

Treatment

Surgery: It is not indicated.

Radiation: Only indicated if the leukaemic deposits develop in the coverings of the brain (meninges), the brain and the spinal cord.

Chemotherapy: It intends to eliminate by killing, the leukaemic cells in the bone marrow and the blood and allow the formation of normal blood cells. Commonly used drugs are:

Adriamycin
Cyclophosphamide
Vincristine
Methotrexate

Bleomycin
Prednisolone

These drugs are given in various combinations, depending upon the severity of the disease and the condition of the patient. The treatment is given in phases. In the first phase, the patient is admitted in the ward. Vincristine and prednisolone are the ideal drugs for killing all the leukaemic cells.

Patient is liable to infection of various sorts and bleeding from different sources during the course of chemotherapy. Care is taken to treat them by blood transfusions, antibiotics, platelet transfusions wherever needed. Chemotherapy also worsens the symptoms already present such as weakness, vomiting, loss of appetite. They are treated symptomatically.

Over 90 per cent of the children get into remission within a month. This means that all or almost all cancer cells in the blood have been killed. Those patients who do not go into complete remission, in them further chemotherapy is given.

Even in the stage of complete remission, patients can develop leukaemia spread and deposits in the meninges, brain and the spinal cord. Radiation over the head, and chemotherapy with methotroxate in the cerebrospinal fluid by injection around the spinal cord (intrathecal) is given.

After this initial phase, even though there are no leukaemic cells in the blood, there may be a few in the bone marrow. To kill them, higher dose of chemotherapy is given. At this stage, the therapy is tolerated better by the patient than it was at the initial phase.

After the disease has been brought under remission and control, maintenance therapy is given in moderate doses so as to kill the remaining collections of leukaemic cells anywhere in the body. This treatment is continued on for about two years, and if the patient suffers no relapse then the treatment is stopped.

If relapse of the disease occurs, it is treated again by chemotherapy. After a relapse, unfortunately, the period of remission becomes less and the prognosis worse.

Prognosis

About half of all children patients having acute lymphatic leukaemia can be cured with the current methods of treatment. The risk of relapse is the greatest in the first two years of treatment, after that it gets progressively less.

Early Detection

Signs & Symptoms	*Investigations*
Tiredness in a child without any cause.	High TLC with immature white blood cells.
Bleeding from gums or other places after slight injury.	Bone marrow biopsy examination.
Frequent fever.	
Enlargement of lymph glands.	
Discomfort or pain over the bones.	
Anaemia.	

Chronic Leukaemias

These are also divided into two types, depending upon the type of white blood cells involved.

1. Chronic lymphocytic leukaemia (CLL).
2. Chronic myeloid leukaemia (CML).

Symptoms

Tiredness
Loss of weight
Loss of appetite
Fever
Pain in abdomen due to enlarged spleen
Occasional bleeding from any source

Diagnosis

This is established by the same methods as they are for acute leukaemias.

Treatment

Surgery: It has no role in the cure of the disease. Sometimes painful enlarged spleen is surgically removed.

Radiation: Radiation over the spleen, reduces its size and also lessens the number of leukaemia cells in the blood.

Chemotherapy: It lessens the symptoms. Busulphan is the drug of choice. Many patients have remission of symptoms for long periods.

Bone Marrow Transplantation in Leukaemias

Bone marrow transplant is the treatment of choice for leukaemia patients of younger age group. The results are good, provided a suitable donor of the bone marrow is available. A sibling is preferable for this purpose. The technique is simple, but great experience is necessary.

Cells from a normal marrow can be given intravenously to a patient who has been specially prepared. These cells go to the marrow and produce enough white and red blood cells and also platelets to restore blood normality in about 3 weeks. It takes longer, months or even years, for the normal bone marrow to stabilize. Bone marrow transplantation thus offers the possibility of replacing diseased with healthy blood tissue.

Supportive Therapy in Leukaemias

This is very necessary particularly in the acute forms of leukaemia.

Anaemia is treated with transfusions of red cell concentrate to maintain an adequate haemoglobin level, preferably above 10 gms per cent. Bleeding is due mainly to diminished platelet count in the blood (thrombocytopaenia) and is exacerbated by infection. Platelet transfusions are required. Platelet transfusion may also be given in anticipation of bleeding in a leukaemia patient with low platelet count in the blood. Infection is a serious and frequent problem. An infection can arise very rapidly within hours and it is necessary to act quickly when it occurs.

Unexplained fever over 38°C, lasting more than 6 hours, should be regarded as due to infection until proved otherwise.

Appropriate antibiotic is given intravenously to control the infection. If it fails to control fever and there is marked diminution of polymorph white cells, then a transfusion of white cells of the blood is given, with very good results.

Prognosis

Control of the disease and symptomatic improvement for a number of years is achieved in most patients, but ultimately an aggressive, untreatable disease develops.

Early Detection

Signs & Symptoms	*Investigations*
Loss of weight in an adult without any visible cause.	High TLC with immature white blood cells.
Loss of appetite.	Bone marrow biopsy examination.
Low-grade fever.	
Pain or discomfort in abdomen due to a mass in the left upper abdomen.	
Occasional bleeding from any source.	
Anaemia.	

10

Lymphomas

These are cancers of the lymph glands. While most cancers occurring anywhere spread into lymph glands, lymphomas primarily involve the lymph nodes. On account of their characteristics, lymphomas are divided into two categories:

1. Hodgkin's lymphoma
2. Non-Hodgkin's lymphoma.

Hodgkin's Lymphoma

The disease is characterized by progressive painless enlargement of lymph glands. It occurs in both sexes, more often in males. Its incidence is low in children, maximum around the age of 20 years, decreases after this age but occurs in older people.

It is distinguished from non-Hodgkin's lymphoma by histological examination of the involved gland, which shows the presence of Reed-Sternberg cells, now thought to be cancer cells.

Cause(s)

It is not known.

Symptoms

Painless swelling of a group of glands, more often on one side of the neck. The involvement of the glands may be present in the thorax or the abdomen.

Loss of weight
Diminished appetite
Feeling of ill health
Fever which comes on and abates, leaving behind increasing weakness.

Diagnosis

Routine: Blood: Hb, RBC, TLC may be normal. DLC may show some increase of eosinophil cells.

Special: Biopsy examination of the involved lymph gland shows the characteristic microscopic picture of Hodgkin's disease, thus clinching the diagnosis.

Additional: X-ray of the chest may show opacities of the Hodgkin's disease if the lung is involved.

Ultrasound examination and CT scan, may show the involvement of the organ such as the liver.

Treatment

Hodgkin's disease is thought to arise in one region of the body and spread from there to others. It is, therefore, important to establish the extent of the disease at the time of diagnosis because staging largely determines the way the treatment is to be given. There are four clinical stages, based primarily on the extent of the disease.

Stage I: Only one group of glands is involved anywhere in the body.

Stage II: More than one group of glands is involved, but only on one side of the body.

Stage III: More than one group of glands are involved, but on both sides of the body.

Stage IV: Besides the glands, there is involvement of the lungs, liver, bones.

Surgery: In stage I, surgery is resorted to, in order to remove the involved lymph nodes.

Radiation: In stage II and III, radiation is the treatment of choice. It is given 4 to 5 days a week, for 3 to 4 weeks. The usual side-effects are nausea, vomiting, tiredness, soreness over the radiated area.

Chemotherapy: When the disease is widespread, only chemotherapy may be of help. Different group of drugs are given.

MOPP: Nitrogen Mustard, Vincristine, also called Oncovin, Prednisolone, Procarbazine.

MVPP: Nitrogen Mustard, Vinblastine, Prednisolone, Procarbazine.

ABVD: Adriamycin, Bleomycin, Vinblastine, DTIC.

The drugs are usually given intravenously and repeated weekly. Tablets are taken by mouth about a fortnight after the injection.

Prognosis

The results of treatment are best in those with a localized disease, discovered early.

Early Detection

Signs & Symptoms	*Investigations*
Painless swelling in a group of glands, more often on one side of the neck.	Raised ESR.
Fever which comes on and abates frequently.	Biopsy examination of the involved lumph gland in the neck or abdomen or other sites.
Loss of weight.	
Loss of appetite.	

Non-Hodgkin's Lymphoma

This comprises all lymphomas other than Hodgkin's. Most of these occur in people above 50 years of age, though some occur in children as well. They differ from Hodgkin's disease because of their different histological picture. These lymphomas grow rapidly, but are potentially curable.

Cause(s)
It is not known.

Symptoms
Lymph node enlargement is the most common presenting finding and is usually painless unless it has developed very quickly. The nodes are discrete and firm. Tissues and organs other than lymph node are involved more often than in the Hodgkin's.

The other symptoms present are:

Tiredness and lassitude.

Loss of weight.

Fever with sweating.

Symptoms also depend on the site where the lymphoma is located. In the chest, there may be breathlessness and coughing; in the abdomen, there may be enlargement of the abdomen, discomfort, pain, obstruction in the intestinal tract or jaundice.

Diagnosis

Routine: Blood: TLC, DLC may be normal, Hb is decreased. ESR is raised.

Special: Biopsy examination of the involved lymph gland clinches the diagnosis.

Additional: If spread in other parts of the body is suspected, then ultrasound examination of the abdomen, or CT of the abdomen or chest, or X-ray of the chest is done.

Treatment
It depends upon the type of lymphoma and its staging. The staging process is similar to that of Hodgkin's.

Surgery: Because the disease is generally widespread, surgery is not helpful.

Radiation: Majority of these lymphomas respond to radiation. The patient may live for many years after treatment, even though the disease is not eradicated.

Chemotherapy: The drugs commonly used are

Cyclophosphamide or Chlorambucil. A combination of drugs called CVP (Cyclophosphamide, Vincristine and Prednisolone) is also useful. The period of treatment may be for up to 6 months.

Response to chemotherapy is good. Some patients live even after ten years.

Radiation and chemotherapy are, many a time, used together, leading to remission of disease for up to even ten years. But the disease does get cured for ever.

For more rapidly progressive lymphomas, the chemotherapy combinations recommended are as follows:

1. Cyclophosphamide, Adriamycin, Vincristine, Prednisolone.

2. Cyclophosphamide, Adriamycin, Prednisolone, Procarbazine Bleomycin, Vincristine.

3. Bleomycin, Vincristine, Methotrexate, Cytosine rabinoside, Leucovorin.

4. Cyclophosphamide, Vincristine, Prednisolone.

Any of these regimes is given intermittently usually at 3-weekly intervals for 6 cycles. Side-effects are nausea, vomiting, tiredness, and increased risk of infection.

Prognosis

The patient may live for over 10 years. Chemotherapy has increased years of survival.

Early Detection

Signs & Symptoms	*Investigations*
Painless lymph gland enlargement anywhere in the body.	Raised ESR.
	Biopsy examination of the involved lymph gland.
Tiredness and lassitude.	
Fever with sweating.	

11

Cancer of the Brain

Brain cancers occur either primarily in the brain itself, or spread to the brain from other sites such as lungs, breasts, lymphomas, leukaemias, etc.

Since the skull provides no scope for expansion, when the cancer mass grows, it causes pressure symptoms on other parts of the brain.

Brain cancers are amongst the commonest cancers in childhood. After the leukaemias, lymphomas and the kidney cancers, they constitute the most frequently encountered cancer in childhood. Approximately 15 to 20 per cent of all brain cancers occur below the age of 15 years.

Brain cancer can arise from any of the different cells that constitute the brain substance. Each cell type may behave differently as regards to symptoms and treatment. The important types of brain cancers are:

1. Medulloblastoma
2. Glioma

In a study reported from All India Institute of Medical Sciences, New Delhi, 419 cases of cancer of the brain in children below 16 years, were seen between the years 1968-1980. There were 7 patients below 2 years of age. The

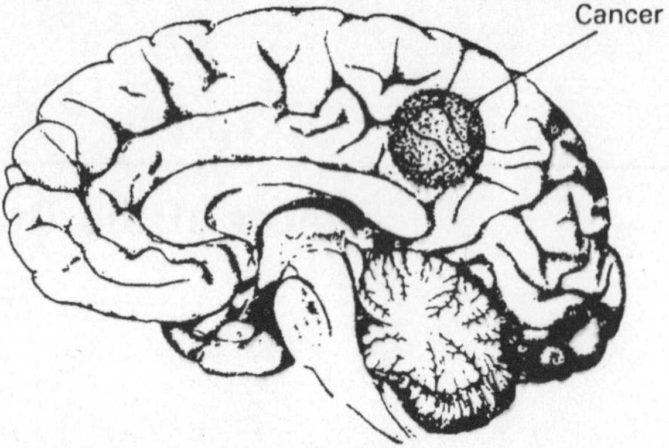

Cancer of the Brain

highest incidence was between 10 to 15 years of age. There was a distinct male preponderance; the male to female ratio being 1.9:1. The male sex predominance was even more marked in cases of ependymoma and medulloblastoma; the ratio reaching 3:1.

Cause(s)
It is not known.

Symptoms
Symptoms depend on the:

1. area involved, and
2. the severity of pressure produced by the cancer mass on other parts of the brain.

Epileptic fits are one of the commonest symptoms.

Headache, nausea and vomiting are the symptoms due to the pressure exerted by the cancer mass.

Other symptoms of loss of function of the involved part vary from case to case.

Diagnosis

Routine: History of the case.

Physical examination.

Blood: Hb,RBC, TLC, DLC, may be normal.

Special: X-ray of the skull may reveal the cancer. CT scan of the brain indicates clearly the site and the size of the cancer, the density may indicate type of the cancer.

Brain scan shows the condensed radioactive material injected into the blood, on to the gamma camera. The cancer tissue shows as an inactive area.

Electroencephalogram (EEG) may indicate the site of the lesion, but not its nature.

The exact nature of the cancer, in the majority of the cases, can only be made out on examination of the tissue at the time of the operation.

Treatment of Glioma

It depends upon the cell-type of the cancer. It is the commonest cancer of the brain. It occurs in the young as well as the old. Some gliomas are faster-growing than the others.

Surgery: Those that are superficial can be easily removed. Before surgery is undertaken, large doses of a steroid dexamethasone (Decadron) are given, so as to drain the fluid out of the cancer mass and so to reduce its size.

The cancer and some part of the normal tissue around it, are removed. After the operation, the symptoms may increase, because of the inflammation caused by surgery, but these symptoms diminish with time.

Radiotherapy: Since it may not have been possible to remove all the cancer cells, radiotherapy is given to kill off the remaining cells. In some cases it effects a cure.

Chemotherapy: Combination of drugs used are:

BCNU

CCNU

The side-effects are modest, but chemotherapy does not make the cure certain.

Treatment of Medulloblastoma

Surgery: The brain tissue involved in the cancer is removed as far as possible and feasible.

Radiation: High dose radiation is given at the site of the cancer mass, and low dosages, all over the brain and the spinal cord. It takes about 6 to 8 weeks.

Chemotherapy: The drug is given intravenously and/or through injection into the cerebrospinal fluid by piercing the coverings (theca) of the spinal cord.

As a result of the combined effect of surgery, radiation and chemotherapy, more than half the children patients live for 5 years or more. Its prognosis is better than that of glioma.

Secondary Brain Cancers

Spread of a cancer from some other part of the body to the brain is commoner than the primary cancer in the brain. The symptoms produced in the brain are the same as with primary, only that the patient is known to have a primary cancer somewhere else in the body.

Diagnosis

Diagnosis of the primary site
Diagnosis of the cancer in the brain

Treatment

Treatment depends on the nature of the primary cancer.

Surgery: It is only done if there is only one secondary in the brain, and the primary has been removed or managed.

Radiation: This is the line of treatment more often adopted. Surgery and radiotherapy can cure or control the disease for many years.

Early Detection

Signs & Symptoms	*Investigations*
Constant and increasing headache.	X-ray of the skull. CT scan of the skull.
Nausea and vomiting.	
Epileptic fit.	
Loss of function of a part of the body.	

12

Cancer of the Thyroid

Thyroid gland is situated in the front of the neck, most of it on the two sides of the larynx. Its secretion pours directly into the bloodstream and regulates among many other things, the metabolism of the body.

The swelling of the thyroid, is more often due to other causes than the cancer, iodine deficiency and goitre being the commonest. Cancer of the thyroid occurs mostly in older people. Its association with chronic thyroiditis particularly Hashimoto's disease is well confirmed.

Cause(s)

It is not known. Its association with chronic thyroid inflammation particularly Hashimoto's disease is well known.

Symptoms

A nodular swelling or a generalized swelling of the thyroid producing prominence of the veins in the neck.

Diagnosis

Routine: Blood: Hb, TLC, DLC, ESR, may be normal.

Special: X-ray of the neck.

Ultra-sound examination of the thyroid to see whether the swelling is solid or contains liquid and so may be a cyst.

Thyroid scan to see whether any area is inactive and so

suspicious of cancer. Needle biopsy of the swelling and its histological examination. This reveals the type of cancer as well.

Additional: X-ray of the chest and suspected bone, to see whether there is spread of the cancer over there.

Treatment

Surgery: The involved part of the thyroid is removed and also the surrounding normal area.

Some part of the normal gland is left intact in order to make available the thyroid secretions needed by the body. Danger to laryngeal nerves is there during surgery, which can make a person hoarse.

Radiation: In cancers, which are very fast growing, radiation keeps in check the growth, and may be the spread of the cancer to other parts of the body.

If the cancer has spread to some part and can be localised, radiation over the area helps to keep in check its growth.

Chemotherapy: The results of chemotherapy are not very satisfactory. Adriamycin helps in only in 20 per cent of the cases.

Prognosis

It is usually a slow-growing cancer, and chances of cure through surgery at an early stage are good. Fast-growing, fast-spreading cancers carry a bad prognosis. An analysis of the post-operative follow-up shows that, on the whole, the prognosis of cancer of the thyroid is good, if treated early and properly.

Early Detection

Signs & Symptoms	*Investigations*
Gradual increase in swelling of the thyroid gland in the neck.	Thyroid scan to see whether any area is inactive and so suspicious. Needle biopsy of the swelling and its histological examination.

13

Cancers of Gastro-Intestinal Tract

Gastro-intestinal tract begins at the mouth and ends at the anus. In between it comprises from above downwards pharynx, oesophagus, stomach, small and large intestine.

The functioning of this system along with its associated organs such as pancreas, gall-bladder and liver is digestion and absorption of food.

Cancer of the Mouth (Oral Cancer)

Cancer of the tongue, mouth and pharynx is much more common in India, Bangladesh, Sri Lanka, Thailand and Indonesia than in other countries. It accounts as much as 30 to 50 per cent of all cancers in India. In the Western countries, it accounts for only 3 to 5 per cent of all cancers.

Causes

Approximately 90 per cent of oral cancers in India can be attributed to tobacco chewing and also smoking. These cancers almost always occur on the side of the mouth where the tobacco quid is kept, and the risk of cancer rises drastically for those who keep the tobacco quid in the mouth over-

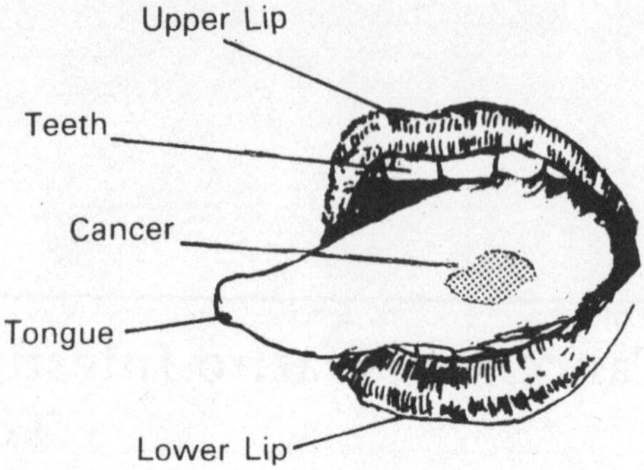

Cancer of the Tongue

night. A link also seems to exist between infection with HSV (Herpes simplex virus) and oral cancer.

Symptoms

Onset of the cancer at this site is usually preceded by the inner lining of the lip turning into a white patch on which a hard mass slowly develops, the top of which some times becomes an ulcer.

Cancer of the lower lip is generally caused by the habit of depositing *khaini*, a mixture of tobacco and lime under the lower lip from where it is chewed slowly. It is seen in the eastern parts of Uttar Pradesh and Bihar.

Cancer of the cheek appears as a hard thickening which is painless. Sometimes an ulcer forms over it. If a painless swelling or an ulcer with a hard base forms and does not heal up in about two weeks, one must consult a competent doctor to rule out cancer.

Chewing or smoking tobacco and the chronic irritation caused by irregular teeth have been suspected to lead to cancer at this site. Cancer of the tongue involves the back of the tongue and at this site grows unnoticed for many months. It then involves lymph glands in the neck which become

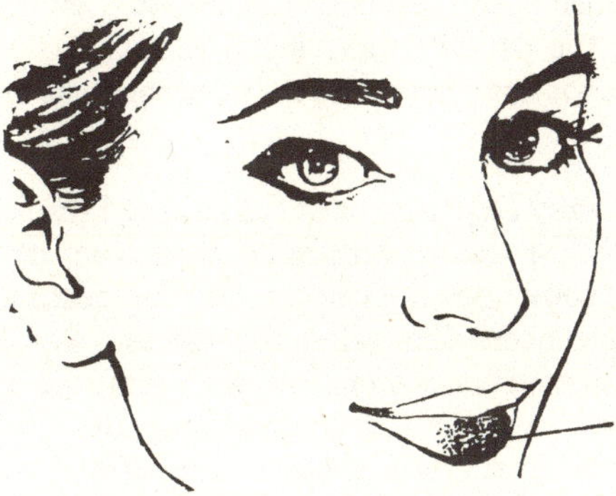

Cancer of the Lower Lip

enlarged and sometimes it is for them that the patient seeks medical advice. This is generally seen more often in men.

Diagnosis

Routine: Physical examination of the local part provides a suspicion.

Blood: Hb, RBC, TLC, DLC, may be normal.

ESR may be raised.

Special: Biopsy examination of the involved part confirms the diagnosis.

Treatment

Surgery: Excision of the involved part, the surrounding areas and the lymph nodes, if involved.

Radiation: It is given when suspicion of spread is present, and the whole of the involved area has not been removed through surgery.

Chemotherapy: It is not of much use.

Prognosis

Presently, more than 50 per cent of oral cancers are detected only after they have reached an advanced stage. Such cancers are disfiguring and painful, the treatment required is both extensive and expensive, and survival rates are low, with less than one-tenth of the patients surviving 5 years.

Surgery and radiotherapy can cure only the early cancers.

Indian Studies

From the Radiotherapy Department of Safdarjung Hospital, New Delhi, in 1987, it was reported that 6 per cent of all the cancer patients coming to the Department for treatment were that of oral cancer. Generally, the disease was far advanced and the survival rates were low with radiotherapy and/or surgery. The treatment with chemotherapeutic drugs was mostly palliative, though their combination with radiation or surgery produced good results in some instances.

In a study reported from Tata Institute of Fundamental Research, Bombay, in 1986, total oral cancer patients numbering 65, could be detected, in a house to house survey of 470,000 villagers in Ernakulam district, Kerala. The average age at the time of diagnosis of oral cancer was 35 years, and 78 per cent were men. The information regarding the tobacco usage was available for 64 patients, and prior to the diagnosis of oral cancer, all of them used tobacco in one form or the other. Even after the treatment of oral cancer, 43 per cent of the patients continued using tobacco, mostly as a smoking habit. More than half of the patients (33 out of 58) were treated less than 5 years before the survey was carried out. This indicated that the survival rate of oral cancer patients was probably not very good.

Early Detection

Signs & Symptoms	*Investigations*
History of chewing tobacco. Non-healing hard-based ulcer can anywhere in the mouth: 1. inside the lower or upper lip 2. on the side of the tongue 3. inside the cheek	Biopsy examination of the part involved.

Cancer of the Oesophagus

Oesophagus is the part of the gastro intestinal tract connecting pharynx of the mouth with the stomach. The lower end of the oesophagus which connects with the stomach normally remains partially closed so as not to allow the acid contents of the stomach to come and injure the oesophagus.

In India, oesophagus is the commonest site of gastro-intestinal cancer after the oral cancer.

Causes

Cancer of the oesophagus is common in Kashmir. Amongst the food habits of Kashmiris which differ from the people in other parts of the country, are consumption of large quantities of very hot saltish tea (*noon chai*), high intake of spices such as chillies, animal fats and smoking. These factors, along with attendant vitamin deficiency, may combine to produce injury of the oesophageal lining, leading to the high incidence of oesophageal inflammation seen in the Kashmiri population.

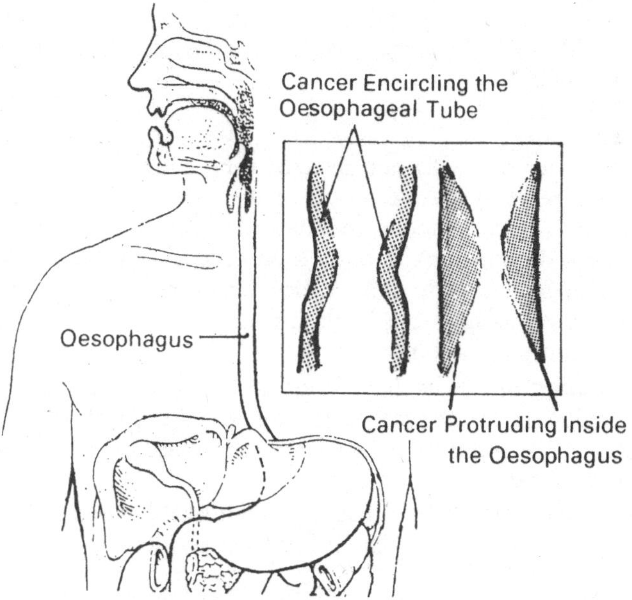

Cancer of the Oesophagus

Symptoms

Difficulty in swallowing solid or semi-solid food and in later stages even liquid food.

Pain in the middle of the chest and also in the back.

Loss of weight.

Vomiting of food that has been taken lately, sometimes mixed with blood.

Diagnosis

Routine: Blood: Hb, and RBC may be lowered.

TLC and DLC may be normal.

ESR is raised.

Stool : Evidence of altered (occult) blood may be seen in the stool examination.

Special: Barium swallow may reveal a cancer or an ulceration.

Endoscopy (oesophagoscopy) may show the lesion directly.

Biopsy examination taken through endoscopic forceps, would clinch the diagnosis.

Additional: Liver scan may reveal if the cancer has spread in the liver.

Treatment

The cancer is usually not detected early enough.

Surgery: Surgical removal of the cancer in the upper two-thirds of the oesophagus is more difficult technically than in the lower one-third. Both the thorax and the abdomen have to be opened, so as to remove the cancer tissue and to rejoin the normal oesophagus with stomach. Healing from the operation takes a long time.

Radiation: It is only done to give some relief for sometime from the symptoms, such as pain or difficulty in eating. It is given for 4 or 5 days each week for a total of about 5 weeks.

Side-effects include nausea, diminished appetite and initially an increase in the difficulty in swallowing.

Surgery and radiation may be given together.

Chemotherapy: No useful drug is available to treat the cancer of the oesophagus or its secondaries if they have spread in the liver, lungs and bones.

Prognosis

Oesophageal cancer has a grim prognosis, as it does not produce clear symptoms early enough. Vague discomfort during swallowing and heaviness or uneasiness underneath the sternum are usually ignored by the patient so that the cancer is not detected early.

Early Detection

Signs & Symptoms	*Investigations*
History of living in a region of the country where this cancer is common. Difficulty in swallowing solid or semi-solid food. Discomfort or pain in the middle of the chest and also in the back. Vomiting of food that has been taken lately, sometimes mixed with blood.	Barium swallow. Endoscopy (oesophagoscopy) which shows the lesion directly. Biopsy examination of the tissue taken through the endoscope.

Cancer of the Stomach

Stomach is the first part of the gastro-intestinal tract where the food stays for some time and gets broken down and digested. If the food contains any substance that is carcinogenic, the stomach is the first part to be affected.

Cause(s)

The cause is not known. Heavy alcohol drinkers suffer from it more. It occurs in the older age-group of people between 50-70 years. Its incidence is highest in Japan.

Symptoms

Symptoms of stomach cancer are very vague to begin with. These are:

Diminished appetite
Loss of weight
Discomfort and pain in the abdomen
Vomit containing blood

Many a time, the only symptom is diminished appetite and not being well.

Diagnosis

Routine: Blood: TLC and DLC may be normal.
Hb may be low.
ESR is raised.
Stool examination may show occult blood in it.

Special: Barium meal may show a filling defect at the site of the cancer growth.

Gastroscopy may indicate the cancer tissue in the wall of the stomach, which can be seen directly by the eye applied to the endoscope introduced inside the stomach.

Gastric biopsy is taken with the help of the forceps of the endoscope, and processed and examined under the microscope. It clinches the diagnosis.

Treatment

Many a time, cancer of the stomach is diagnosed at such a

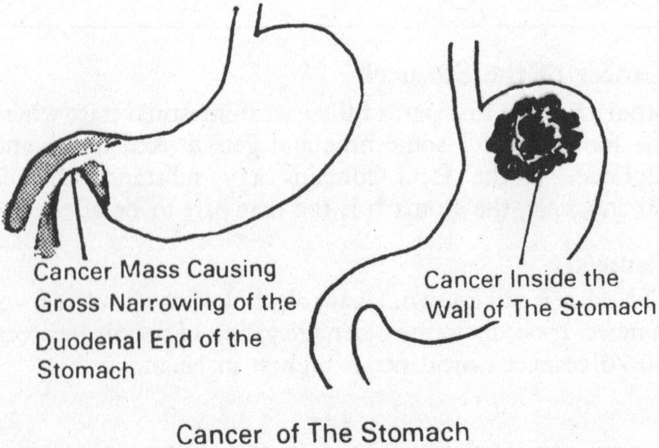

Cancer of The Stomach

late stage that anything that is done is of no help to the patient.

Surgery: Surgery is sometimes undertaken to remove the obstruction, and thus to provide relief to the patient for some time.

If detected early, removal of the involved part and also a large part of the surrounding organ plus all the locally draining lymph glands, (radical gastrectomy) is done, with some degree of success.

After recovery, the patient should take small meals at a time, though more number of times. The food should be well balanced, nutritious and contain very little fibrous part.

Since stomach wall forms vitamin B_{12}, removal of a large part of the stomach, creates its deficiency, so that the patient needs to take it regularly.

Radiation: Radiation therapy is not effective for stomach cancer. However, if the cancer has spread into the surrounding and nearby areas and organs, radiation may provide some relief from pain.

Chemotherapy: A combination of 5-Fluorouracil Adriamycin or Mitomycin is effective, to an extent. 20 to 25 per cent of the patients respond to this line of treatment, but the survival is not much prolonged.

In case of a small local tumour detected early, surgery along with chemotherapy with 5-Fluorouracil is helpful without causing much of side-effects.

Early Detection

Signs & Symptoms	*Investigations*
Diminished appetite. Loss of weight. Discomfort or pain in the abdomen. Vomit containing blood.	Barium meal may show up the cancer. Endoscopy (Gastroscopy) shows the lesion directly. Biopsy taken through endoscopy and its examination reveals the diagnosis.

Cancer of the Colon and Rectum

Large bowel forms lower 1.5 metre part of the gastro-intestinal tract, going up from the right lower abdomen as ascending colon, then horizontally as transverse colon, coming down on the left side as descending colon and then as rectum ending at the anus.

Cancers of the colon and rectum are not common in India. But they are one of the most common sites of cancer in the USA, Denmark and some other European countries. In the USA nearly 45,000 people die of this cancer.

Causes

Those people who pass stool daily or even oftener because of having more roughage in the diet, have less of cancer of the large bowel. Those who form and pass less stool because their diet contains no roughage, have a higher incidence of colon cancer. This might be due either to the longer staying in of the cancer-causing diet, or the production of bacteria due to putrefaction of faecal matter which may be carcinogenic.

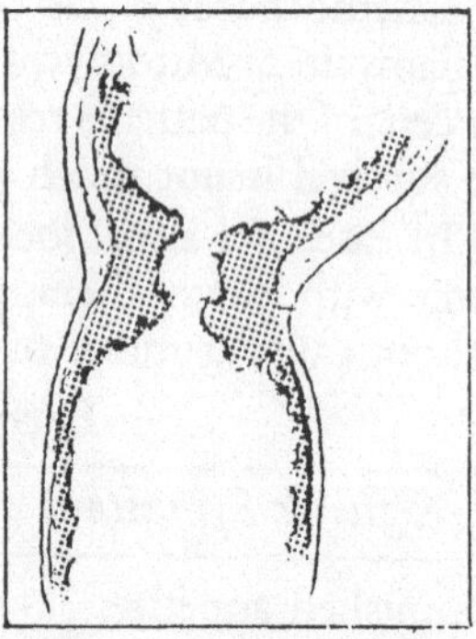

Cancer Mass Causing Gross Narrowing of the Large Bowel

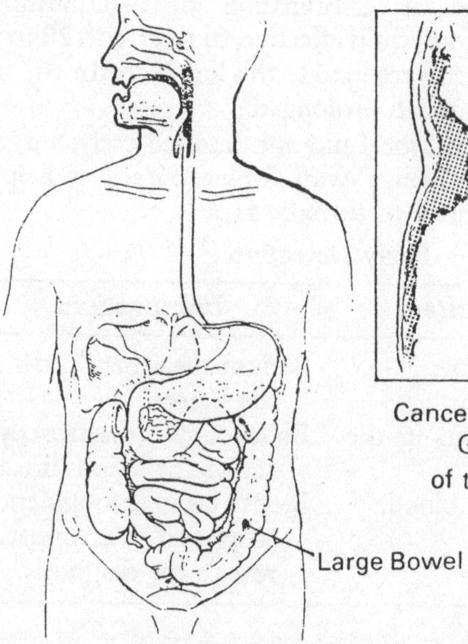

Cancer of the Large Bowel

Symptoms

Constipation or diarrhoea alternating with each other.

Pain in the lower abdomen.

Blood in the stool.

Early fatigue.

Loss of weight.

Diagnosis

Routine: Blood: Hb, RBC, TLC, DLC may be normal. ESR may be raised.

Stool shows blood in it.

Special: Sigmoidoscopy and biopsy examination or colonoscopy and biopsy, confirm the diagnosis.

Additional: Ultrasound scan of the liver for secondaries. X-ray of the chest for secondaries.

Treatment

Surgery: Chances of removal of the cancerous part are good with surgery, depending upon the extent to which the cancer has spread. If it is confined to the inner lining of the colon (stage I), the chances of cure are excellent. If it has spread in the muscular wall of the colon, the chances are fair. But if the cancer has spread into the lymph glands draining from the area of cancer, then even in spite of the removal of the involved lymph glands, the chances of cure are diminished.

If the cancer involves the rectum then after removal of the involved part, instead of connecting the normal colon with the anus, the surgeon opens the end of the normal colon on to the abdomen. The faecal matter collects in a bag tied over the opening and is removed and cleaned periodically. This procedure is called colostomy. It is inconvenient but the patient gets used to it.

Radiation: If the cancer is in the sigmoid colon or the rectum and gone on to stage II or III, then radiation before or after surgery, is helpful, in lessening the chances of relapse.

Chemotherapy: About 20 per cent of the patients repond to 5-Fluorouracil. The drug does not cause much of side-effects.

This drug is also used if secondaries of the cancer have developed in other parts of the body.

Early Detection

Signs & Symptoms	*Investigations*
Constipation or diarrhoea alternating with each other.	Sigmoidoscopy and biopsy examination.
Pain in the lower abdomen.	Colonoscopy and biopsy examination.
Passing blood in the stool.	
Loss of weight.	

Cancer of the Liver

Liver is present on the right side of the upper part of the abdomen, just under the diaphragm. Its main function is to convert the digested food into integral parts of the body. The cells of which it is made up, are very special cells to perform their function, and have the capacity to regenerate themselves also.

The commonest disease of the liver in India is infectious hepatitis or common jaundice.

Cancer of the liver may be primary, that is, arising from the liver itself or secondary, i.e. arising from another organ (matastasis) and spreading to the liver. The incidence of the primary cancer of the liver shows great geographical variations, being common in Africa and South East Asia and India, and less common in Western countries. It occurs predominantly in males, and in 80 per cent of the cases, the patient already has cirrhosis of the liver.

Causes

A liver which has developed cirrhosis because of an earlier attack of infectious hepatitis due to Hepatitis B virus or excessive intake of alcohol, is more liable to develop primary cancer.

Presence in the food of some chemical substances such as Aflatoxin, which occurs particularly in ground-nuts infected with the fungus called Aspergillus fumigatus is also known to cause cancer. In the majority of the cases, however, the cause cannot be pin-pointed.

Symptoms

Loss of appetite

Weakness

Discomfort or pain, sometimes very severe in the upper abdomen.

Swollen abdomen due to rapid enlargement of the liver and/or the presence of fluid in the abdomen, a condition called ascites.

Diagnosis

Routine: Blood: Hb and RBC may be low.

TLC and DLC may be normal.

ESR is raised.

Special: Liver function tests show impairment.

Liver ultrasound and CT scan give the outline of the liver and its consistency, and so give an idea about the nature of the disease.

Liver biopsy taken through a fine needle and its examination, gives the exact nature of cells and the diagnosis.

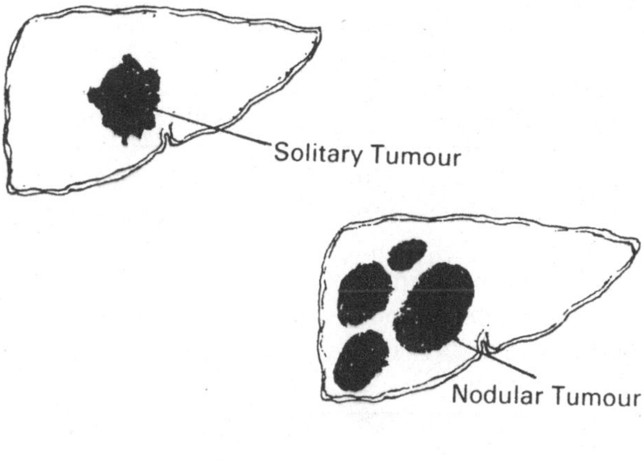

Cancer of the Liver

In view of its simplicity, it is recommended in all cases suspected of the disease.

Treatment

Surgical: If the liver cancer is discovered very early and is very small in size and localized, it is possible to remove it surgically. In most other cases, surgery is of no help.

Radiation: It only helps sometimes in relieving some symptoms, such as pain, for sometime only.

Chemotherapy: It does not help.

Prognosis

The patient of liver cancer, may die within a year.

Secondary Cancer in Liver

Spread of cancer in the liver secondary to the initial occurrence of cancer in some other parts of the body, is a very common occurrence. Secondaries in the liver usually originate from cancers in the bronchus, breast, abdomen or pelvis. They may be single or multiple. Peritoneal dissemination frequently results in ascites.

In patients presenting with advanced cancers, secondaries in liver are present in 30 to 50 per cent of the cases. Average survival of the patient ranges between 2 to 6 months. Surgery and radiation are unhelpful. Isolated good responses may be obtained by chemotherapeutic drugs.

Early Detection

Signs & Symptoms	*Investigations*
History of having had jaundice earlier in life or of heavy drinking. Discomfort or pain sometimes severe, in the upper abdomen. Swollen abdomen.	Needle biopsy of the liver and its examination.

Cancer of the Gall-bladder

Diseases of the gall-bladder are commoner in females than males. Gall-bladder cancer occurs in older age-group people.

Cause(s)

It is not known. A diseased gall-bladder having gall-stones which irritate its wall may make it more liable to develop cancer.

Symptoms

The symptoms are vague. Abdominal discomfort, or pain in the upper abdomen or under the right ribs. These are:

Indigestion.
Loss of appetite.
Loss of weight.
Jaundice in the later stages.

Diagnosis

Routine: Blood: Hb, RBC, TLG, DLC may be normal.

Special: Cholecystography

Ultrasonoscopy of the gall-bladder.

Biopsy examination after opening the abdomen surgically, confirms the diagnosis.

Treatment

The patient usually presents herself/himself in the later stages of the disease when it has infiltrated and spread in the surrounding areas. Hence, the cure is usually not possible. Vague symptoms lead to late diagnosis.

Early Detection

Signs & Symptoms	*Investigations*
History of having had gall-bladder disease.	Ultrasonoscopy of the gall-bladder.
Vague discomfort in upper right abdomen.	Biopsy examination after opening up the abdomen.
Loss of appetite.	
Loss of weight.	

Surgery: It may be of some help, only in the early stages.

Radiation: It can lessen the symptoms and keep the disease under control for some time.

Chemotherapy: It is given, but is not curative.

Cancer of the Pancreas

Pancreas lies in the abdomen between the lower border of the stomach and the upper border of the duodenum, the first part of the small intestine. It produces digestive enzymes which pass into the duodenum by a duct to digest the food. Special type of cells of the pancreas, produce insulin which is absorbed into the blood and helps in keeping in balance the level of the blood sugar.

Cancer of the pancreas occurs in older people of both the sexes.

Cause(s)

It is not known.

Symptoms

Pain in the upper abdomen, and also sometimes in the back.

Loss of weight.

Loss of appetite.

Jaundice in the later stages.

There may be no symptoms at all, till the cancer has spread into the adjoining tissues and then produce symptoms because of that.

Diagnosis

Routine: Blood: Hb, RBC, TLC, DLC may be normal. ESR is raised.

Special: Barium meal may show narrowing of the duodenum if the pancreas is enlarged and pressing upon it.

Ultrasound examination may show the cancer mass in the region of the pancreas.

CT scan may show the cancer mass in the region of the pancreas.

Endoscopy, including ERCP allows direct vision of the pancreatic duct and the bile duct.

Many a time, all the above tests, do not confirm the diagnosis, and opening the abdomen and seeing the organ and the area around and the biopsy examination establishes the diagnosis.

Treatment

Surgery: If the cancer is detected early and is small, confined to the pancreatic duct only, surgical removal is done.

More often the cancer has spread into the adjoining areas and also obstructed the bile duct in the duodenum or the duodenum itself. Then surgery is performed only to remove the obstruction so as to remove jaundice.

Radiation: It can only work to the extent that it may reduce the size of cancer and reduce the obstruction, if present.

Chemotherapy: It has only limited role 5-Fluorouracil is the most frequently used drug either singly or along with Adriamycin and Mitomycin C. Most of the patients do not respond favourably; some do.

Prognosis

Cure is only rarely possible in pancreatic cancer because of the advanced stage when detected. Only relief of symptoms is obtained by even the combination of approaches.

Early Detection

Signs & Symptoms	*Investigations*
Pain in the upper abdomen, sometimes going to the back. Loss of appetite. Loss of weight.	Barium meal may show narrowing of the duodenum if the pancreas is enlarged and pressing against it. Ultrasound and CT scan may show the cancer mass in the pancreatic area. Endoscopy including ERCP allows direct vision of the pancreatic and bile ducts, and may show up the cancer.

14

Cancer of the Lung

Lungs are the two organs in the chest which transfer oxygen that we breathe in into the blood, and breath out the CO_2 generated in the body. Cancer of the lungs is categorised depending upon the type of cells involved. The two categories are:

1. Small-cell cancer.
2. Non-small cell cancer.

Small-cell cancer grows and spreads fast in the body. About one-fourth of all lung cancers are of this type. It is also called oat-cell cancer, because its cells, under the microscope, look like oat grains. This type is not much associated with smoking.

Non-small cell cancer has under it three varieties:

1. Squamous or epidermoid.
2. Adenocarcinoma.
3. Large cell cancer.

Squamous cell cancer is the one which is associated with tobacco smoking. All these three varieties grow less rapidly than the small cell cancer and hence their treatment is more or less on similar lines.

Lung cancer accounts for more than 50 per cent of all

male deaths from cancer in the Western countries where it is widely prevalent. Of all deaths from lung cancer, small cell carcinoma accounts for 25 per cent, squamous for 50 per cent, large cell 10 per cent and adenocarcinoma 10 per cent.

Lung cancer arises from bronchial epithelium or mucous glands and at an early stage may occlude the bronchial lumen. When the cancer mass obstructs a major bronchus, it causes collapse of the lung.

A tumour arising from a peripheral bronchus may attain a very large size without producing a significant degree of collapse.

It may involve the pleura either directly or by lymphatic spread, causing a pleural effusion which is often blood-stained. It may also extend into the chest wall and cause severe pain. The cancer or its lymph node metastases may extend into the mediastinum, the space between the two lungs in the chest. The incidence of lung cancer in India is about 4 per cent of all cancers.

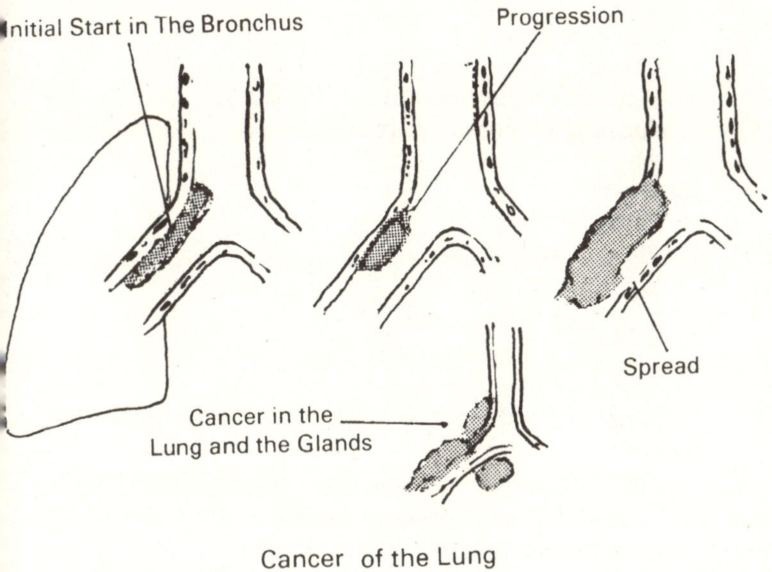

Cancer of the Lung

Causes

After the Second World War, the incidence of lung cancer has sharply increased in developed countries. In England and Wales, the death rate is continuously increasing—having risen to 37.5 deaths in males and 5.8 deaths in females per 100,000 population in 1975.

Cancer of the lung particularly squamous cell type, has increased in incidence all over the world where the tobacco is smoked, in particular, tobacco in the form of cigarettes. The risk of getting cancer of the lungs is increased in accordance with the number of cigarettes smoked. Those who leave smoking, lessen the risk of getting lung cancer.

Symptoms

Cough, sometimes with blood in the phlegm
Fever
Loss of appetite
Loss of weight
Hoarseness of voice sometimes
Pain in the chest
Breathlessness
Clubbing of the finger nails

Metastasis to the brain are commonest from lung cancer, producing a variety of symptoms.

Diagnosis

History taking
Physical examination
Routine: Blood: Hb may be decreased
TLC may be increased
In DLC, polymorphs may be increased
ESR is raised

X-ray of the chest, many a time, indicates suspicion of cancer

Sputum examination for cancer cells is sometimes helpful

Special: CT scan can reveal the presence of cancer in the lung, as well as its spread in the glands.

Fine needle aspiration biopsy examination may establish diagnosis.

Bronchoscopy may show the presence of cancer in the bronchi. A punch biopsy taken from a suspicious site and examined histologically, can reveal the true identity of the lesion. Bronchial aspirate examination histologically, may reveal the nature of the lesion.

Additional: In case there is suspicion of the presence of cancer secondaries in other organs such as liver, bones or brain, an ultrasound examination of the liver, or CT scan of the other organs can reveal the diagnosis.

Treatment

It depends upon the stage of the disease and also on the cell-type of the cancer.

Surgery: In small-cell type cancer, by the time the diagnosis is made, it has already spread all over the body, hence surgery is of no use.

In non-small cell types, if the cancer is small, and localized and has not spread to the regional draining glands, the chances of cure are high. But, unfortunately, a majority of the cases present late. This is because most smokers regard coughing as a usual practice, and many doctors are also beguiled by the fact that coughing is a common symptom in smokers.

If the cancer mass is large and it has spread in the glands or other parts of the body, then even if operation is performed, it is done mainly to lessen the symptoms and not for cure.

Radiation: In small-cell type cancers, it can be used only over some parts of the body where the cancer has spread, and this also for treating the symptoms and not for cure. The same is the case for non-small cell type cancers.

Chemotherapy: In small-cell type cancers, the drugs used are:

Adriamycin
Cyclophosphamide
Vincristine

While symptoms of the disease may decrease for sometime, the side-effects produced such as malaise, nausea, vomiting, hair loss, risk of increased infection, are real hazards. Only relief from troublesome symptoms may be achieved for sometimes but not the cure.

Prognosis

Since most of the cases of lung cancer, present themselves when the cancer has spread from the lungs to the glands or other parts of the body, the cure is difficult.

Countries where `quit smoking', compaigns have succeeded, are showing lesser incidence of cancer. The best preventive is not to smoke.

Secondary Tumours of the Lung

Blood borne metastatic deposits in the lungs may be derived from primary cancer almost anywhere in the body. The secondary deposits are usually multiple and blateral.

Early Detection

Signs & Symptoms	*Investigations*
History of smoking for many years.	X-ray chest may indicate cancer.
Cough, sometimes tinged with blood.	Bronchoscopy for direct vision of cancer.
Loss of appetite.	Bronchoscopy for biopsy and its examination.
Loss of weight.	
Fever.	
Hoarseness of voice, sometimes.	
Pain in the chest.	
Breathlessness.	
Clubbing of the finger nails.	

15

Cancer of the Breast

Breast cancer is common. It usually occurs in women past the age of 40 years, though it has been seen to occur earlier as well. The incidence of breast cancer in India is reported to be 20 per 100,000 women. It occurs a decade earlier than in the Western women; the mean age of occurrence is about 42 years in India, as compared to 53 years in the white women.

Incidence of breast cancer is higher in the Western countries than it is in India. Different studies have shown the incidence there per 1,00,000 women as follows:

USA	71.4	Denmark	49.1
Switzerland	70.6	England	48.0
Israel	55.5	Yugoslavia	28.3

In Japan, the incidence is less than India, viz. 13.0/100,000 women.

Cause(s)

It is not known. The major known determinants of risk for breast cancer are delayed age at first pregnancy, family history of breast cancer, giving of oestrogens, fibrocystic breast disease, and exposure to the ionizing radiation.

Symptoms

A lump or nodule in the breast.

As this lump grows, it gets attached to the skin of the breast.

Lymph nodes become enlarged and papable in the axilla on the side of the disease.

Diagnosis

Routine: Physical examination of the patient and palpation of her breast to see whether the nodule is attached to the overlying skin, which it does in cases of cancer.

Blood: Hb, RBC, TLC, DLC may be normal.

Special: Taking out the lump of the breast surgically or if it is a big one, a part of it, and its histological examination, is necessary to establish a diagnosis. Biopsy can be taken under a local anaesthetic or a general one.

Fine needle aspiration biopsy has also been useful not only in differentiating cancer from non-cancer lesions, but it can

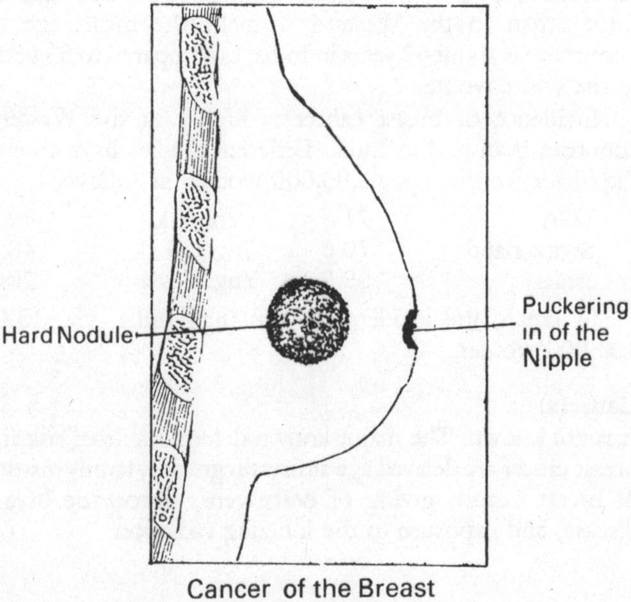

Cancer of the Breast

also pin-point the exact histologic type of the cancer. The overall accuracy was found to be 84.2 per cent in a study, reported from PGI Chandigarh, in 1979.

Treatment

Surgery: If detected early, surgery may bring about a cure. The whole of the breast is removed including the underlying glands. The operation is called radical mastectomy. This is done in order to leave no doubt about recurrence of the cancer.

Radiation: If the cancer mass is of moderate size, then besides the above-stated surgery, radiation treatment is given to the patient in order to kill any remaining cancer cell. Radiation is given 4 to 5 times a week for 4 to 6 weeks. The side-effect of radiation is soreness or discomfort to the exposed area. Radiation is also given in case of recurrence of the disease.

Chemotherapy: In order to do away with exigency of recurrence, chemotherapy is given, besides the surgery and radiation, particularly in younger patients. In older patients, after menopause, the rapidity of growth of the cancer decreases, or the effect of recurrence are slow to appear. A single drug or a combination of them are suggested.

Side-effects include:

Nausea.
Tiredness.
Partial hair loss.
Susceptibility to infection.

Hormone Treatment: It is long known that removal of the ovaries, lessens the size of the breast cancer. The same result can be obtained if the adrenal glands are removed.

Nowadays, instead of doing the operation of removing the ovaries (oophorectomy), anti-hormone drugs like Timoxifen are given in selected patients who are known to respond to such a treatment. Not all patients respond to this treatment; prior testing can reveal which patient would respond.

Indian Studies

In a study reported from Tata Memorial Hospital in 1983, intensive multi-drug post-operative chemotherapy for high risk stage II breast cancer was given. 20 patients (15 pre-menopausal and 5 post-menopausal) with carcinoma of breast involving 4 or more ipsilateral axillary lymph nodes and primary lesions measuring more or equal to 3 cm by 3 cm received 6-monthly cycles of an intensive chemotherapy regime comprising Vincristine, Adriamycin, Cyclophosphamide, Methotrexate and 5-Flourouracil. The surgery done was modified radical mastectomy with axillary glands removal. Post-operative radiation was not given and chemotherapy was instituted within the first 4 weeks of surgery. The treatment was well-tolerated except for marked hair loss and stomatitis. Fifteen patients (75 per cent) survived recurrence-free for 12 to 36 months with a median of 24 months. Two patients developed early recurr-ence in chest wall in 7th and 10th months of post-operative period. The other 3 patients developed distant organ and bone metastases in 14th, 17th, and 18th months after the surgery.

Prognosis

If the breast cancer recurs, after any or all modes of treatment, the chances of cure, are not bright. However, even such a patient can live for many years. An older patient may live up to her normal life span.

Early Detection

Signs & Symptoms	*Investigations*
A lump or nodule in the breast.	Fine needle aspiration biopsy and its examination. Taking out the lump and its histological examination.

16

Cancer of the Genito-Urinary System

These two separate systems of the body have been grouped together here for the convenience of description. *Genito* pertains to reproduction and *urinary* to formation and excretion of urine.

Cancer of the female genitals particularly the uterus and its cervix is very common in India, in fact, one of the commonest in the females.

Cancer of the Uterine Cervix

Cervix is the last part of the uterus which protrudes slightly into the vagina.

Cancer of the uterine cervix is common in Indian women, accounting for 25 to 50 per cent of all cancers in women seen in hospitals in different parts of India. Figures published in 1980 showed that in Guntur (Andhra Pradesh), cervical cancer accounted for 61.5 per cent, in Vishakhapatnam (Andhra Pradesh) 71.8 per cent, in Vellor (Tamil Nadu) 54.5 per cent, and in Calcutta 23.3 per cent, of all cancers in females. Cancer cervix is also widely present in countries of the South East Asia region.

Incidence of and mortality from cervical cancer has

declined in Western countries considerably in recent decades. Hygienic measures, early detection by cervical cytology and effective treatment have contributed to this significantly.

Cause(s)

Cervical cervix may have multiple causes. Important risk factors include poor genital hygiene, early marriage, early coitus, multiple sexual contacts and repeated childbirth. It is rare in nuns. On the other hand, prostitutes have a very high incidence of cancer cervix. Another observation is that cancer cervix is more common in the lower socio-economic groups than in the higher socio-economic groups, reflecting probably poor genital hygiene.

Symptoms

Vaginal discharge mixed with blood.

Bleeding in between periods or after the sexual act.

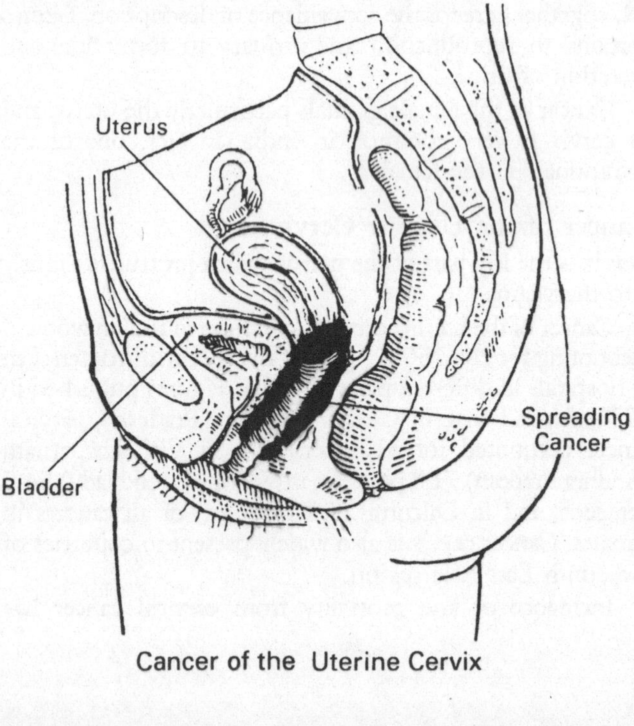

Cancer of the Uterine Cervix

Diagnosis

Routine: Physical check-up of the local part.

Blood: Hb may be low.

TLC may show rise.

DLC may show increase in polymorphs; this is due to infection.

ESR is raised.

Special: PAP smear test of the surface of the cervix is a must. This by itself can make the diagnosis of cancer. It can also detect the impending cancer, by seeing cells, which though not cancerous, yet are likely to become so.

A biopsy of the cervix is done and examined to confirm the diagnosis.

Treatment

It depends on the stage of the disease at the time of presentation to the doctor.

Surgery: If cancer has involved only the surface of the cervix, surgical removal of the cervix and the uterus provides complete cure. If the cancer has infiltrated the wall of cervix, either surgery or radiation is done. Mostly, either of them provide a cure. If the cancer has spread beyond the cervix, into the surrounding tissue or organs, surgery has no role.

Radiation: It is done in stage II, III, and IV of the cervical cancer. Radiation is given both externally as well as internally, by implantation of the radium needles into the cancerous area.

Radiation has many side-effects, such as infertility and early menopause, scarring and drying of the vagina, causing difficulty during intercourse and irritation of the bladder.

Chemotherapy: It has not proved very effective.

Prognosis

Detected and removed surgically in the earliest stage, it can be cured.

Prevention

PAP test in all women going to a gynaecologist is a must.

Early Detection

Signs & Symptoms	*Investigations*
Vaginal discharge mixed with blood.	PAP smear test from the surface of the cervix.
Bleeding in between periods or after the sexual act.	Biopsy examination of the involved part of the cervix.

Cancer of the Uterus

Uterus present in the lower part of the abdomen, is the organ where the foetus normally resides during pregnancy.

Uterus is very much liable to develop, hard, roundish masses in its walls, which also protrude into cavity of the uterus, and cause excessive bleeding. They may be present more than one at a time. They are called fibroids and they are not cancer.

Cancer of the uterus is quite common in females in India. In Bombay, Dr. Jussawalla (1973) found its incidence to be 25.1 per 100,000 females.

Cause(s)

It is not known. It occurs later in life.

Symptoms

Bleeding from the vagina at times other than the menstruation.

Vaginal discharge.

Diagnosis

Routine: Physical examination of the local part.

Blood: Hb may be decreased.

TLC may be raised and so also the polymorph count, due to infection.

ESR is raised.

Special: Through the procedure of dilatation of the uterus and its curettage (D&C) the uterus is slightly dilated, and a curettage introduced and scrubbed against the lining, (endometrium). The cells that come out in the bleeding are examined histologically for cancer.

Abdominal ultrasound and CT scan of the abdomen is done to gauze the site and size of the cancer.

Treatment

It depends upon the stage ot the disease. Many a time, surgery, radiation and chemotherapy, are all used.

Surgery: If the cancer is yet confined to the uterus and has not spread out, surgical removal of the uterus, the fallopian tubes and the ovaries (hysterectomy with bilateral salpingo-oophorectomy) is done. The results are good in 90 per cent of the cases.

Radiation: If the cancer has spread further, extensive surgery as well as radiation are given. The results are good in only 50 per cent of the cases. Radiation is given from outside source, as well as implantation of radiation needles in the cancer mass so as to kill the cancer cells.

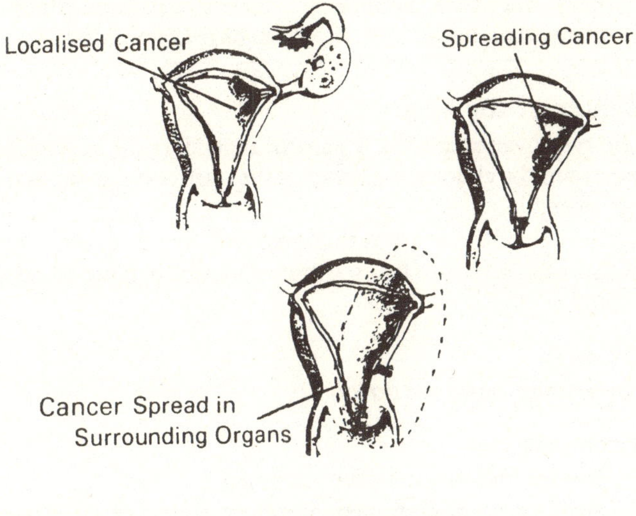

Cancer of the Uterus

Chemotherapy: Progesterone, a female hormone, is helpful in reducing the size of cancer in about 30 per cent of the cases. This is given in advanced cases of cancer, along with all the other treatments.

Anti-cancer drugs are also given in cases where there is suspicion that all the cancer has not been removed.

Prevention

There is mounting evidence of a steady rise in the incidence of uterine cancer in India. It was supposed to be confined to the post-menopausal age group, but now it is seen with increasing frequency in middle-age and early-age groups. The diagnosis of cancer in its pre-invasive stage is clearly the key to the control of uterine cancer.

Early Detection

Signs & Symptoms	*Investigations*
Bleeding from the vagina at times other than the time of menstruation.	Biopsy taken of the inner uterine wall and its histological examination.

Cancer of the Ovary

The two ovaries are the organs of reproduction in females present in the abdomen. Cancer of the ovaries occurs in older age group.

Cancer of the ovary is the most fatal female cancer, one of the reasons for this being that it cannot be diagnosed early enough.

Cause(s)

No definite cause is known.

Symptoms

Discomfort in the lower abdomen.

Swelling of the abdomen, due to the spread of the cancer and presence of fluid.

Loss of weight.

Occasional shortness of breath due to presence of fluid in the pleura.

Diagnosis

Routine: Blood: Hb, TLC, DLC, ESR may be almost normal.

Special: Ultrasound examination of the abdomen and pelvic region may show an enlargement of the involved ovary.

CT scan also may show an enlarged ovary. If fluid is present in the abdomen, a little of it is taken for examination for the presence of cancer cells.

Substances produced by cancer cells of the ovary and circulating in the bloodstream are used for diagnosis of the condition. These substances called 'markers', are carcinoembryonic antigen (CEA), Alpha-fetoprotein (AFP), Human chorionic gonadotrphin (HCG) and an enzyme Lactate dehydrogenase (LDH). They are found to be increased in ovarian cancer. Estimation of them can help establish diagnosis.

Diagnosis can only be clinched by opening the abdomen and seeing the organ and by biopsy examination.

Treatment

The type of treatment given depends on the stage of the disease.

Surgery: The chance of cure is high with surgery alone in stage I, when the disease is confined to the ovary only. Both the ovaries, the fallopian tubes, as well as the uterus are removed.

Radiation: If the cancer has entered into stage II (i.e. it has spread beyond ovaries but is confined in the pelvic region), after surgery radiation is given with fair chance of success. Radiation is also given in stage III and IV but the chances of success are not much.

Chemotherapy: This is given in stage II to IV of the disease. A group of drugs called alkylating agents are given with a good response. These drugs usually given by mouth are taken for two to three weeks each month, for several months, even years.

The side-effects are not much. Some centres give a combination of drugs. The drugs used are:

Adriamycin
Cyclophosphamide
Chlorambucil
Cisplatin
Hexamethyl melamine
5-Fluorouracil
Methotrexate

Prognosis

Survival is best in stage I or II of the disease.

Early Detection

Signs & Symptoms	*Investigations*
Discomfort in the lower abdomen.	Ultrasound and CT scan of the ovary.
Loss of weight.	Opening the abdomen and examination of the biopsy taken.

Choricarcinoma or Cancer of the Placenta

It is cancer of the placenta, the tissue that links foetus with the uterus of the mother during pregnancy. It is a rare cancer.

Cause(s)

It develops from an abnormality of the placenta called hydatidiform mole. This cancer of the placenta spreads very quickly in all parts of the body. It may show itself in the mother after abortion or miscarriage or pregnancy.

Symptoms

Continued vaginal bleeding after delivery.
Abdominal pain.
Cough due to spread of the cancer in the lungs.

Nervous system symptoms due to spread in different parts of it.

Diagnosis

Routine: Blood: Hb, TLC, DLC, ESR may be normal.

Special: Increase in the level of human chorionic ganodotrophin in the serum.

Additional: X-ray of the chest, for locating the spread of cancer over there.

CT scan of the brain for the spread of cancer in the brain.

Treatment

Surgery: It has no role.

Radiation: It has no role.

Chemotherapy: It can cure the cancer. Methotrexate is the drug of choice. Even if the cancer has spread in all parts of the body, it can be cured with it.

Early Detection

Signs & Symptoms	*Investigations*
Continued vaginal bleeding after delivery.	Increase in the level of human chorionic gonado-trophin in the serum.

Cancer of the Testes

Not all enlargements of the testes are cancerous. More often it is epidedymitis, inflammation of the tubes, leading to and from the testes, or even presence of fluid in the pouch around the testes, the condition called hydrocele, that causes an enlarged testes.

Cancer of the testes occurs in younger men between the years of 15 to 40.

Cancer of the testes are mainly of two types:

1. Seminoma
2. Teratoma

Seminoma

Cause(s)

It is not known with certainty. Failure of the testes to descend completely from the abdomen where it is situated in the foetus, to the scrotum, is one of the known causes.

Symptoms

It is a malignant tumour of the testes, appearing as a swelling, often painless, in the scrotum.

Occurs in age group of 30 to 40 years.

Enlarged and painful testes.

Spread occurs into the lungs.

Diagnosis

Routine: Blood: Hb, RBC, TLC, DLC, ESR may show no change.

Special: Needle biopsy of involved testes and its examination establishes the diagnosis.

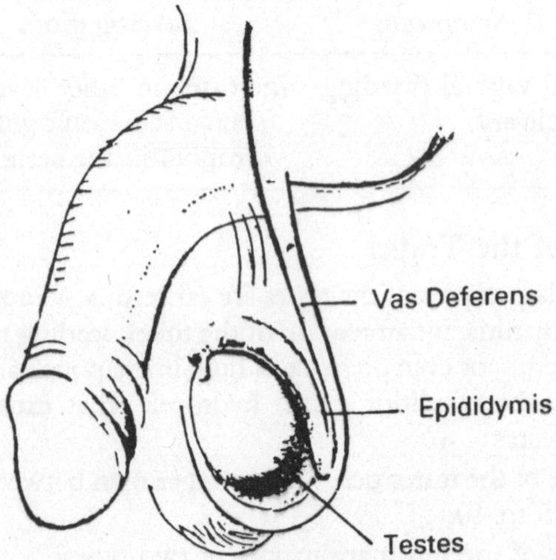

Testes (Normal)

Additional: Ultrasound and CT of the liver and lungs indicate whether the cancer has spread in these organs.

Treatment

Depends upon the stage of the disease:

Stage I: Cancer confined to the testes.

Stage II: Cancer has spread in the lymph nodes in the abdomen.

Stage III: Cancer has spread further and invade the abdomen, liver and lings.

Surgery: Removal of the testes, if in stage I, may cure the disease.

Radiation: If the stage is I or II, radiation is done over the lymph nodes in the abdomen, 4 to 5 exposures a week for 3 to 4 weeks. Cure rate is over 90 per cent.

Chemotherapy: Stage III cancer needs extensive surgery of the parts involved and radiation, as well as chemotherapy.

Teratoma

This tumour spreads from the testes via the lymph channels as well as the bloodstream.

Cause(s)

It is not known.

Diagnosis

Routine: Blood: Hb, RBC, TLC, DLC, ESR may be normal.

Special: Increased levels of Human chorionic gonadotrophin (HCG) and Alfa fetoprotein (AFP), which are produced by this cancer, are increased.

Needle biopsy examination for cancer cells can confirm the diagnosis.

Additional: X-ray chest and CT scan of the lungs, to see if the cancer has spread there.

Blood tests to measure liver and bone marrow function. If the function is deranged, it indicates the spread of cancer over there.

Treatment

Staging is more or less similar to that of seminoma.

Surgery: Removal of the testes and the extensive removal of the lymph glands from the abdomen, cures over 90 per cent in stage I and over 80 per cent in stage II.

Radiation: Radiation is given to the lymph glands in the abdomen in all stages of the disease.

Chemotherapy: It is used in stage II and III. High doses or a combination of drugs like Cis-plastin, Bleomycin and Vinblastine, cure a high percentage of cases. Side-effects of chemotherapy are fairly large. These are:

Feeling of fatigue.
Nausea and vomiting.
Loss of hair.
Damage to the lungs and subsequent breathlessness.
Increased risk of infection.

Prognosis

Detected early, the cure rate is high.

Early Detection

Signs & Symptoms	*Investigations*
Enlarged and painful testes in a man between 20 to 40 years old.	Needle biopsy examination.

Cancer of the Prostate

Prostate, a chestnut shaped gland, encircles the upper-most part of the urethra as it connects with the urinary bladder in the male. Prostate cancer accounts for 16 per cent of all cancers detected in males. It is uncommon among men under forty, but it is the third highest cause of male cancer deaths in men over fifty-five and the leading cause of cancers among men over seventy-five.

Cause(s)

It is not known.

Symptoms

Prostate cancer has to be differentiated from benign prostatic enlargement which is quite common in the same age-group or a little younger, and causes almost the same sort of symptoms. The usual symptoms of benign hypertrophy are:

Hesitancy at the start of passing urine.

Increased frequency of passing urine.

Getting up at night also to pass urine.

Retention of urine.

Men who get cancer of the prostate carry the disease with them for many years without suffering any noticeable symptoms. 90 per cent of the cases are not detected until the cancer has metastasized beyond the prostate gland.Indeed, often the condition is not discovered until an autopsy is performed after death from some other cause. An estimated 15 to 20 per cent of men over fifty may unknowingly be suffering from prostate cancer.

The prostate cancer has in addition to above symptoms of benign hypertrophy,

Pain on passing urine

Blood in urine

Pain in the lower back, pelvis or upper thighs.

Diagnosis

History of symptoms and indicative of the disease.

Routine: Rectal examination for prostate enlargement and irregularity of its surface and complaint by the patient of pain at the site, while doing the examination.

Blood: Hb, RBC, TLC, DLC, ESR may be normal.

Special: A needle biopsy taken through the rectal examination and its histological examination may clinch the diagnosis.

Serum estimation of acid phosphatase, which is increased in prostate cancer.

Additional: Prostate cancer may first reveal itself in the bones as metastasis or secondaries. X-ray of the bones can reveal this condition. Isotope scan of the suspicious bones can be done.

Treatment

Surgery: It is done in cases where the cancer is confined to the prostate and the patient is somewhat younger and in good health. Sexual potency is usually lost after it.

Radiation: 50 to 70 per cent cases survive for 5 years after radiation and also retain their sexual potency. Survival with surgery or radiation is almost similar. Radiation is used when the cancer has spread out of the gland, but has not involved the bones.

Surgery and radiation both together are also used.

Hormone Therapy: Giving oestrogen, the female sex hormone, or removal of the testes of the patient, slows the rate of growth of the cancer and as well reduces its size. This treatment provides relief from pain in the bones, and removes obstruction in passing urine, both of which symptoms are very troublesome for the patient. Hormone treatment, however, does not cure the cancer.

Chemotherapy: This is not of much use.

Prognosis

The chance of cure is best when the cancer is confined to the prostate and is removed surgically.

Early Detection

Signs & Symptoms	*Investigations*
Non-cancer prostate enlargement causes. Hesitancy to start passing urine. Increased frequency of passing urine. Prostate cancer in addition to above, causes. Pain on passing urine. Blood in the urine.	Needle biopsy examination of the prostate provides an early diagnosis.

Cancer of the Penis

Cancer of the penis is a frequent male cancer in all races which do not practice circumcision. Its incidence is highly variable: it is rare among Jews anywhere. It accounts for less than one per cent of male cancers in the United States.

Cause(s)

Poor hygiene of the inside of the skin that covers the glans penis, seems to be one of the causes.

Symptoms

A hard-base chronic sore that does not heal and infiltrates and grows.

Diagnosis

Routine: Blood: Hb, RBC, TLC, DLC, ESR may be normal.

Special: Biopsy from the area involved and its histological examination confirms the diagnosis.

Treatment

Surgical: Amputation of the part involved, as well as of the tissues that could have been involved.

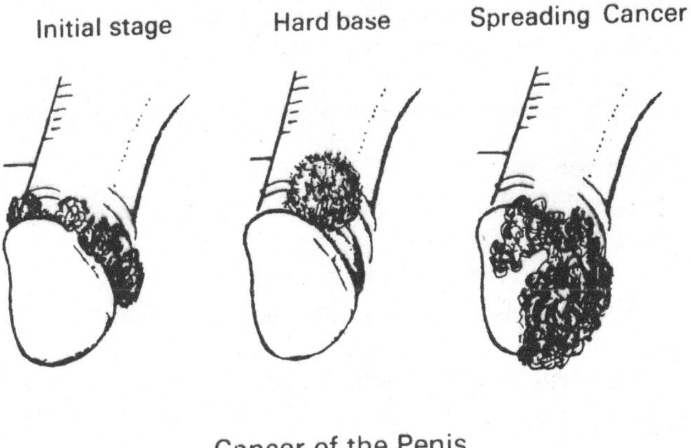

Cancer of the Penis

Radiation: Not very helpful. It may decrease the size of the glands in the groin that are involved.

Chemotherapy: It is of no use.

Prognosis

If diagnosed early and surgical amputation done before it has spread in the adjoining area and lymph glands, the prognosis is good.

Early Detection

Signs & Symptoms	*Investigations*
A hard-base chronic ulcer on the penis that does not heal, but spreads into the tissues around.	Biopsy examination of the involved area, provides early diagnosis.

Cancer of the Urinary Bladder

Cancer of the urinary bladder occurs mostly in older people of both the sexes. It is easy to detect and difficult to cure.

Cause(s)

It is not known. Aniline dyes and other chemicals in the industry are known to cause cancer at this site.

Symptoms

Increased frequency in passing urine.
Blood (haematuria) in the urine.
Pain on passing urine.
Pain in lower abdomen when the cancer has spread.

Diagnosis

Routine: Blood: Hb, RBC, TLC, DLC, ESR may not reveal any abnormality.

Urine: RBC may be present.

Special: Microscopic examination of urine may reveal cancer cells.

Intravenous pyelography is done to see the whole of the urinary tract, including the bladder. Cystography is done so as to directly visualize the inside of the urinary bladder, which may reveal the cancer.

Additional: Bone scan and liver ultrasound is done to see if the cancer has spread to these organs.

Treatment

Surgery: Endoscopic resection of the cancer if the cancer has involved only the inner lining. The surgeon after passing the cystoscope, can resect the cancer mass.

Bladder cancers are usually widespread, and unless there is only one tumour, this is not resorted to.

Radiation: It is usually combined with surgery. This is useful, particularly:

1. When there are wart-like growth, on the inside surface of the bladder.
2. When there is widespread cancer, not completely removable by surgery and the patient is in pain.

Chemotherapy: Single or a group of drugs are tried:

Adriamycin
5-Fluorouracil
Methotrexate
Thiotepa
Cisplatin

These drugs are effective but cause side-effects.

Prognosis

The chances of survival depend very much on the extent of the cancer spread and the stage at which the patient presents.

Early Detection

Signs & Symptoms	*Investigations*
Increased frequency of passing urine. Blood in the urine.	Cystoscopy for direct vision of the inner surface of the bladder. Biopsy taken through cystoscopy and its examination.

Cancer of the Kidney

The two kidneys present in the abdomen, clean the blood of the various harmful metabolic products such as urea, creatinine, and keep a balance of water and other electrolytes in the body.

Cancer of the kidney are:

1. Hypernephroma
2. Wilm's tumour

Hypernephroma is found in adults and older age-group people. Wilm's tumour occurs more often in children.

Hypernephroma

Cause(s)

It is not known. Smokers suffer from kidney cancer five times more than the non-smokers. Some chemicals used in the industry also can cause it. It occurs more often in males, after the age of 50 years.

Symptoms

General ill health in the early stages.

Loss of weight.

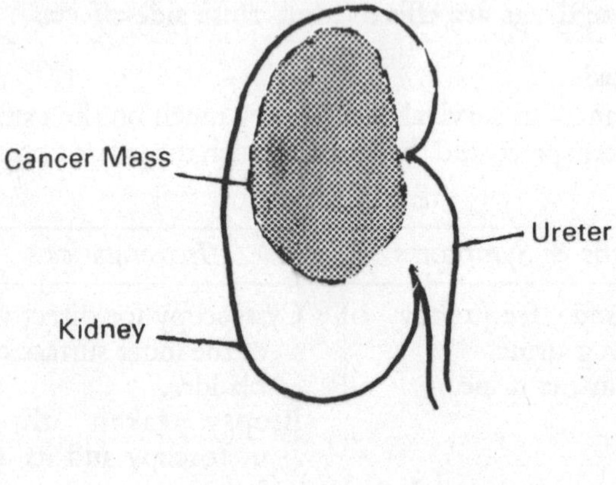

Cancer of the Kidney

Loss of appetite.
Blood in urine.
Fever of unexplained origin.
Pain in the abdomen.

Diagnosis

Routine: History taking.

Blood: Hb, TLC, DLC, ESR may show no significant change.

Urine : Usually shows presence of red blood cells in it.

Special: Ultrasound scan of the kidney.

CT scan of the kidney.

Intravenous pyelogram.

Fine needle aspiration biopsy of the kidney and its examination for cancer cells establishes the diagnosis.

Additional: Bone scan and lung X-ray and scan, to see if the tumour has spread in these parts.

Treatment

Surgery: If the tumour has not spread beyond the kidney, removal of the diseased kidney can cure the patient. The other normal kidney can look after the function of the both.

Radiation: If the cancer has spread to bones or other parts, radiation may relieve symptoms.

Hormones: In advanced cases of cancer, giving female sex hormone progesterone, or male sex hormone (androgen) may help in reducing the size of the cancer.

Chemotherapy: It is not helpful.

Prognosis

The outlook is variable. Sometimes spontaneous remissions occur. At other times, the patient may continue living for years.

Wilm's Tumour

It is a cancer of the kidney, occurring more often in children between the ages of 1 to 5 years.

Cause(s)

It is not known.

The children who suffer from this cancer, often have partial or complete absence of the iris of the eye-balls, have abnormalities of the urinary system, i.e. in kidneys, ureters or the bladder.

Symptoms

A firm irregular, non-tender lump in the abdomen.

Abdominal discomfort.

Blood in the urine.

Fever.

Loss of appetite and weight. Sometimes it is discovered accidentally by the patient. Blood in the urine occurs late in the disease.

Diagnosis

Routine: History taking

Blood: Hb, TLC, DLC, ESR may show no change.

Urine : Presence of red blood cells.

Special: Plain X-ray of the abdomen.

IVP of the kidneys.

Ultrasound of the abdomen.

CT scan of the abdomen.

Fine needle aspiration biopsy of the kidney, establishes diagnosis.

Additional: X-ray chest and bones.

CT scan of the chest, liver and suspected bones, to locate the spread of cancer.

Treatment

Surgery: It is the treatment of choice for a cancer which is still localized to the kidney. Removal of the involved kidney, provides a cure.

Radiation: It is usually given after the operation, when it is suspected that the complete removal of the cancer has not been possible.

Chemotherapy: This treatment is given along with radiation in cancer suspected to have spread around. Actinomycin-D has been given successfully in these cases. Adriamycin and Vincristine have also been used lately with good results. Chemotherapy is started soon after the surgery and is continued on intermittently for a period up to 15 months.

Prognosis

The chances of cure are the best in children under 2 years of age, where the cancer is still confined to the kidney. Up to 80 per cent of the patients get cured after chemotherapy treatment.

Early Detection

Signs & Symptoms	*Investigations*
Pain in the abdomen. Fever. Loss of weight. Presence of blood in the urine.	Ultrasound and CT scan of the kidney. Fine needle aspiration biopsy of the kidney and its examination.

17

Neuroblastoma

It arises from the cells of the sympathetic nerves and in the adrenal glands. These nerves are spread over all parts of the body. The cancer occurs more commonly in the abdomen. The cancer spreads rapidly in the body through the blood vessels as well as lymphatic channels. The cancer cells produce a substance called catecholamine which raises the blood pressure.

This is a common cancer of childhood, forming 10 per cent of all cancers occurring in this age group.

Symptoms

Lump in the abdomen.

Weight loss.

Diminished appetite.

Swelling in the neck.

Protrusion of the eyeball, due to the occurrence of the cancer behind the eyeball.

Diagnosis

Routine: Blood: HB, RBC, TLC, DLC may be normal. ESR is raised.

Serum catecolamines are increased.

Special: Biopsy examination from the involved part confirms the diagnosis.

Additional: X-rays of the chest, abdomen, suspected bones are taken to look for the spread of the cancer.

Treatment

Surgery: If the cancer is localized and can be taken out completely, then this is the method of choice and cure rate is over 90 per cent.

If the cancer has spread, partial removal of the cancer would not help much.

Radiation: Radiation is given over the cancer which cannot be removed through surgery. The cancer is very amenable to radiation and so only low dosages are given.

Chemotherapy: If the cancer has spread, besides radiation, a combined drug chemotherapy with a group of drugs is given, to improve the results. It does not, however, bring about a cure.

Prognosis

The younger the age, say 1 to 2 years, the better the chances of cure.

Early Detection

Signs & Symptoms	*Investigations*
Lump in the abdomen, or protrusion of an eyeball in a child.	Biopsy examination of the involved part.
Diminished appetite.	
Loss of weight.	

18

Cancer of the Muscles (Rhabdomyosarcoma)

Cancer of the muscles can occur anywhere in the body. It is easy to diagnose because it is present in the superficial surfaces of the body, such as the extremities and the abdomen. It is not a common cancer.

Cause(s)
It is not known.

Symptoms
They depend on the site of the cancer. A lump may appear in muscle, arm, leg or neck. This lump does not appear after an injury and does not disappear, but gradually increases in size.

Diagnosis

Routine: Blood: Hb, RBC, TLC, DLC, ESR may show no change.

Special: A biopsy examination of the lump confirms the diagnosis.

Additional: If the cancer has infiltrated deeper or spread in other parts of the body, the following investigations may be needed:

CT scan of the suspected bone.
CT scan of the abdomen and chest.
Ultrasound or CT scan of the liver.

Treatment

Help is taken, frequently, of all the modes of treatment.

Surgery: Surgical removal of the involved part, if localized, may provide a cure.

Radiotherapy: High doses of radiotherapy are given to the area from where the cancer had been removed. It is given for 4 to 5 days a week, for 4 to 8 weeks.

Chemotherapy. It is given along with surgery and radiation. The drugs more often used are a combination of the following:

Actinomycin D
Vincristine
Cyclophosphamide
Adriamycin

This group of drugs is given at 3-weekly intervals.

Prognosis

Depends upon the site of the cancer. If it is superficial and detected at an early stage, the treatment has more than 50 per cent chance of cure.

If the cell of the cancer is on the maturer side, it has better prospects than that of the immature cells.

Younger children have better chance of survival.

Early Detection

Signs & Symptoms	*Investigations*
A lump in the muscle that has not appeared after injury, and it increases in size.	Biopsy examination of the lump.

19

Cancer of the Bone

Cancer of the bone occur both in the young and the old, in males and females. This cancer is of various types. The common among them are as follows:

1. Osteogenic Sarcoma.
2. Ewing's Sarcoma.
3. Multiple Myeloma.

Osteogenic Sarcoma

This cancer occurs predominantly in males between the ages of 10 to 25 years. Any bone may be involved.

Cause(s)

It is not known.

Symptoms

Pain and tender swelling of the bone and the tissues around it.

Loss of weight.

Fatigue.

Involved bone may break without much of an injury.

Spread may occur in the lungs and bones.

Diagnosis

Routine: Blood: Hb, TLC, DLC may show no change. ESR may be raised.

Special: X-ray of the bone which shows destruction of the bone at the site of the cancer.

Bone biopsy establishes the diagnosis of cancer and also the type of cancer.

Additional: In order to look for the spread of the cancer, the following tests are done:

X-ray of the chest.

Liver scan.

Treatment

Surgery. This involves amputation of the long bone much above the cancer site.

Many cases of spread of the cancer to other parts are seen even after the surgery.

Radiation. Radiation is given before the surgery in some centres, in order to shrink the tumour or to eliminate it.

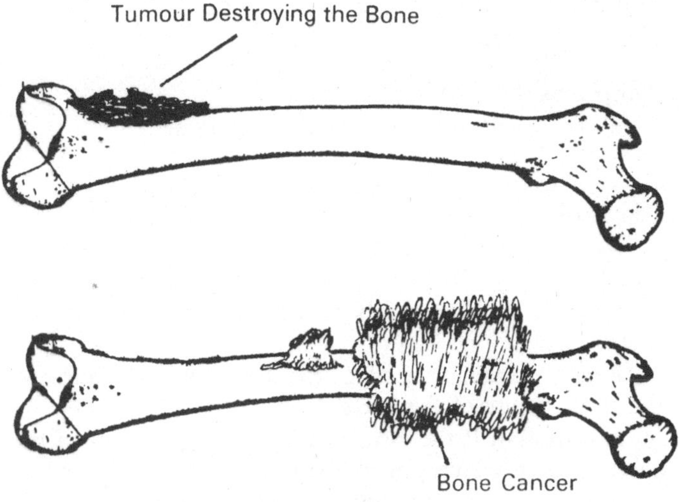

Cancer of the Bone

Chemotherapy: Most centres use chemotherapy after surgery and radiation to kill the metastases which even though small may have yet occurred. The drugs commonly used are:

Methotrexate
Adriamycine
Vincristine
Cyclophosphamide

The treatment is given intermittently for 1 to 2 years. If an obvious spread has occurred in the lungs or bones, surgical removal is attempted, and then chemotherapy given.

Prognosis

If detected when localized, the chances of cure after surgery, are above 50 per cent. Some osteogenic sarcomas are slow-growing; in them the chances of success are 70 to 80 per cent.

Ewing's Sarcoma

This is a tumour of the bones, occurring in children, more often boys, between the age of 5 to 15 years. It may involve any bone of the body.

Cause(s)

It is not known.

Symptoms

Continuous and increasing pain over a bone.

Swelling of a bone.

Diagnosis

Routine: Blood: Hb, TLC, DLC are normal. ESR is raised.

Special: X-ray of the bone which shows swelling and destruction.

Biopsy examination of the involved bone which shows the exact nature of the cancer.

Additional: If the cancer has spread, then X-ray of the chest is taken which can confirm it.

Bone scan of the other suspected bones is done.

Ultrasound examination of the liver is done to look for the secondaries.

Treatment

Surgery: This is unhelpful.

Radiation: In high doses, it is given over the diseased area 4 to 5 days a week for 6 to 8 weeks. Soreness and reddening and later thickening of the skin occurs as a side-effect.

Chemotherapy: Chemotherapy is indicated when the cancer has spread to other parts of the body.

The drugs most commonly used are:
Vincristine
Cyclophosphamide
Adriamycin
Actinomycin D
Treatment is given intermittently for some months.

Prognosis

Two decades back, Ewing's sarcoma was described as the most lethal primary cancer of the bone, reported 5-years survival being 0 to 12 per cent. Availability of new chemotherapeutic agents has, however, changed the picture. Initial trials were limited to single agent chemotherapy with Cyclophosphamide, Vincristine, Melphalan and 5-Fluorouracil with some improvement. Addition of drugs like Adriamycin, Actinomycin D, Bleomycin, and CCNU have changed the picture for the better dramatically. With such chemotherapy, 5-year survivals are reported to be around 70 per cent.

Radiation and chemotherapy together can cause a cure in case the cancer is localized and has not spread in other parts. In cases where the cancer has spread, this treatment prolongs life and lessens suffering.

Multiple Myeloma

This is cancer of one of the cells called plasma cell of the bone marrow and occasionally of the soft tissues. Plasma cell normally produces antibodies. When this cell becomes cancerous, it cannot produce those antibodies, with the result that the patient is very susceptible to infections.

This cancer is very uncommon under the age of 30 years. It becomes increasingly frequent thereafter, having its peak incidence between 60 and 70 years. Males are involved rather more frequently than females. There is a long pre-clinical phase, in some instances up to 25 years, the disorder being discovered incidentally by laboratory tests during this phase. The patient may thereafter be observed for years before symptoms appear.

Cause(s)
It is not known.

Symptoms

Fatigue
Loss of weight
Fever
Recurrent infections
Bone fractures

Symptoms usually reflect bone involvement, impairment of immune function, kidney damage and anaemia. The diffuse osteoporosis and local erosion of bone by myeloma cells results in stress, pain and eventual pathological fracture. The stress pain is often wandering, difficult to locate and described as rheumatic. On the other hand, the first intimation of trouble may be the sudden onset of acute localized pain due to pathological fracture. These symptoms arise mainly in weight-bearing bones, the vertebrae, pelvis and femur being particularly susceptible. Collapse of a vertebra is common and produces severe nerve root pain. Weight-lifting may also cause pain in arms. Patients are often severely crippled. The progressive impairment of immune function due to the deficiencies of normal immunoglobulins and the excess of abnormal immunoglobulins, render these patients susceptible to infection, particularly of the respiratory tract. Pneumonia is quite frequently the presenting illness and often the cause of death.

Diagnosis

Routine: Blood: Hb and RBC may be markedly decreased. TLC and DIC may be normal. ESR is markedly raised.

Urine shows proteins in it, of a particular variety called Bence-Jones proteins.

X-ray of the involved bone shows typical punched out cavities.

Special. Bone marrow biopsy examination confirms the diagnosis.

Additional. X-ray of the chest and bones are taken for locating the spread of the cancer in these areas.

Treatment

Surgery: It is of no use.

Radiation: It relieves pain in the bones effectively.

Chemotherapy: The commonly used drugs are Melphalan and Prednisolone. This course of treatment is given every 4 to 6 weeks.If this has failed, a group of drugs is given.

Prognosis

After chemotherapy, most of the patients, live longer for many years and comfortably.

When chemotherapy becomes ineffective, patient is treated only for the relief of symptoms.

Early Detection

Signs & Symptoms	*Investigations*
Pain and swelling of a bone or bones and areas around.	Biopsy examination of the involved bone.
Bone fracture without injury.	
Loss of weight.	
Low-grade fever.	
Anaemia.	
Fatigue.	

Cancer of the Skin

Skin cancer is not common in India. It is more common in fair-skinned people. Two main varieties of skin cancers are:

1. Squamous Cell Cancer
2. Malignant Melanoma

Squamous Cell Cancer (Rodent Ulcer)

Cause(s)

Prolonged exposure to direct sunlight in fair-skinned people. It is commonly seen on the skin of the face and the hands.

Symptoms

It appears as an ulcer on the skin with raised margins. This ulcer does not heal with usual antibiotics, etc. The spread of this cancer is slow and long delayed.

Diagnosis

Routine: Blood: Hb, RBC, TLC, DLC, ESR may be normal.

Special: Biopsy from the lesion is taken and examined for cancer cells.

Treatment

Surgery. Excision of the cancerous tissue along with some of the normal one.

If the tumour has spread and gone to the draining lymph glands, these have also to be removed.

Radiation: It may be necessary if the cancer has spread, so as to kill the remnant cells.

Prognosis

Since the cancer is detected early, the cure-rate is over 90 per cent.

Malignant Melanoma

This cancer of the skin is fast growing, and spreads locally and in the regional lymph glands also.

Cause(s)

It occurs both in the parts exposed to the sun, as well as those not thus exposed.

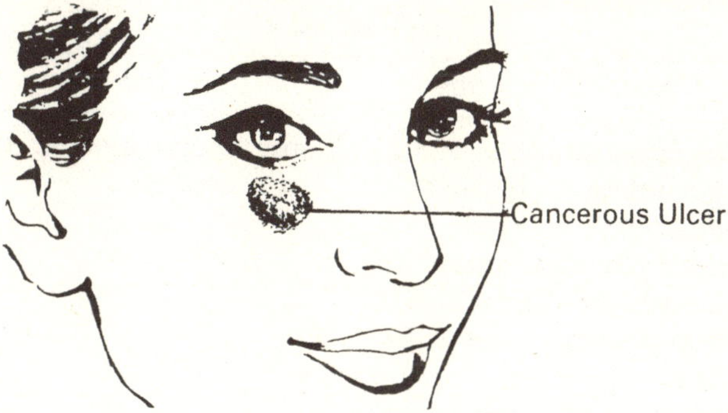

Cancer of the Skin

Symptoms

Sudden growth in a mole or a birthmark.

Bleeding from a mole, or what looks like a mole.

Formation of new moles, around an old one.

Diagnosis

Routine: Blood: Hb, TLC, DLC, ESR may show no change.

Special: Biopsy of the suspected area and its examination for cancer cells.

Additional: X-ray chest and bone scan for secondary spread of the cancer.

Treatment

Surgery. Excision of the cancerous area along with that of the normal skin around it.

Excision of the draining lymph nodes, if suspected of spread.

Radiation. It is more often used for recurrent cases of this cancer.

Chemotherapy: It is not very helpful.

Prognosis

It is good, if the cancer is detected and treated early.

Early Detection

Signs & Symptoms	*Investigations*
Skin ulcer that does not heal, but infiltrates in the area around. Sudden growth in a mole or a birthmark in the skin. Bleeding from a mole in the skin. Formation of new moles around an old one.	Biopsy examination of the part involved.

APPENDIX

Common Anti-Cancer Drugs and Their Characteristics

1. Generic/Trade Names : *Adriamycin* ADRIAMYCIN (Walter Bushnell)

To be given	*Dose*	*Indications*	*Contra-indications*	*Side-effects*
Intravenous injection (I/v)	1.2 to 2.4 mg/kg body weight or 60 to 75 mg/square meter of body surface, given as a single dose every 3 weeks by slow I/v injection.	Used in the treatment of Lymphomas, leukaemias, soft tissue & bone sarcomas.	Liver or heart disorders.	Nausea & vomting, loss of hair.

2. Generic/Trade Names : *Melphalan* ALKERAN (Wellcome)

Orally or injection	Continuous therapy with 2 to 5 mg daily dose, or 7-day course of 10 mg daily. Another course not until the restoration of leukocytes & platelets.	Multiple myeloma, Breast cancer	Low WBC counts; Concurrent radiation therapy	Increased risk of infection, Increased bleeding tendency, Infertility.

3. Generic/Trade Names : *Methotrexate* BIOTREXATE TABLETS/INJECTION (Biochem), NEOTREXATE TABLETS (Biddle Sawyer)

Tablets, Injection I/v or I/m	20 to 40 mg/sq.m. body surface, twice weekly I/v or I/m. Maintenance dose, 15 to 30	Lymphoblastic leukaemia; Choriocarcinoma.	Severe anaemia Diminished WBC. Withdraw the drug for 2 weeks if	Increased risk of infection; Increased bleeding tendency; Sore mouth.

To be given	*Dose*	*Indications*	*Contra-indications*	*Side-effects*
	mg/sq.m. 1 to 2 times a week.		there is severe fall in WBC. Diminished platelets; Pregnancy; Lactation; Kidney and liver diseases.	
4. Generic/Trade Names : *Bleomycin* BLEOCIN (Khandelwal)				
I/v or I/m	30 mg twice weekly, 15 mg daily to 15 mg weekly.	Cancer of the brain, oesophagus, lungs & uterine cervix; Lymphoma	Do not mix glutathione with bleomycin either in I/v infusion or in the syringe. Not to be given during pregnancy.	Fever and shivering; Hair loss; Skin pigmentation and thickening; Lung damage if given in excess.
5. Generic/Trade Names : *Cisplastin* CISPLATIN (Biochem)				
I/v	10 to 80 mg total, or as required.	Cancer of the testes, ovaries, brain, neck & bladder.	Hypersensitivity to the drug, Kidney damage, Patient should be tested repeatedly for ear function.	Nausea & vomiting; Diarrhoea; Increased risk of infection; Increased bleeding tendency; Loss of hearing; Kidney damage, if enough water is not taken.

6. Generic/Trade Names : *Cyclophosphamide* CYLOXAN (Biochem), ENDOXAN-ASTRA (Khandelwal)				
Orally or I/v	50 to 200 mg daily	Hodgkin's disease Leukaemias Multiple myeloma	First three months of pregnancy; Bone-marrow depression; Treatment to be stopped if WBC falls below 3000; Acute urinary tract infection	Nausea and vomiting; Increased frequency of passing urine; Loss of hair; Infertility; Sore mouth; Increased risk of infection; Increased tendency to bleeding.
7. Generic/Trade Names : *5 Fluorouracil* FIVE FLURO (Biddle Swayer), FLURACIL (Biochem)				
Orally or I/v	10 to 15 mg per kg./body-wt. I/v for 5 days, followed by 7.5 mg/kg., alternate days. 4 capsules, alternate day 6 doses	Gastro-intestinal; tract cancer; Breast cancer; Pancreatic cancer	Pregnancy; Bone-marrow depression	Increased risk of infection; Nausea and vomiting; Hair loss; Sore mouth; Increased bleeding tendency.
8. Generic/Trade Names : *Florofur* FURATOR (Biochem)				
Orally	800 to 1200 mg daily in 2 to 4 doses	Cancer of the breast	Pregnancy; Bone-marrow depression	Nausea and vomiting Bone-marrow depression.
9. Generic/Trade Names : *Chlorambucil* LUKERAN (Wellcome)				
Orally	As directed by physician	Lymphomas	Not within 4 weeks of radiation; Low WBC; Low platelet count; Not to be given during pregnancy.	Increased bleeding tendency; Increased risk of infection; Infertility.

10. Generic/Trade Names : *L-Asparaginase* LEUNASE (Biochem)

To be given	*Dose*	*Indications*	*Contra-indications*	*Side-effects*
I/v	50 to 200 KU per kg. body-wt. or every alternate day I/v	Acute laukaemia; Lymphoma	Hypersensitivity to the drug	Fever; Sleepiness; High blood sugar

11. Generic/Trade Names : *6 Mercaptopurine* PURINETHAL (Wellcome)

Orally	As prescribed by the physican	Acute leukaemia	Pregnancy; Kidney disorders	Increased risk of infection; Increased bleeding tendency.

12. Generic/Trade Names : *Mitomycin-C* MITOMYCIN-C Kyoma (Biochem)

I/v	6 to 10 mg I/v twice daily 0.05 mg per/kg body wt. daily for 5 days, total dose 60 to 100 mg	Adenocarcinoma Lymphosarcoma Seminoma	Bone-marrow depression; Bleeding tendency	Increased risk of infection; Bleeding tendency; Nausea and vomiting; Hair loss.

13. Generic/Trade Names : *Mustine* MUSTINE Hcl (Boots)

I/v	0.1 mg per kg body wt. daily for 3 to 4 days, not to exceed 8 mg in a single dose. To be given I/v in 500 ml of normal saline	Hodgkin's diseases; Chronic leukaemia; Lung cancer	Early pregnancy. To be given strictly intravenous, second course not be given before 6 weeks.	Nausea and vomiting; Bleeding tendency; Hair loss.

14. Generic/Trade Names : *Vincristine* VINCRISTINE (Biochem), NEOCRISTIN (Biddle Sawyer), RICRISTIN

To be given	*Dose*	*Indications*	*Contra-indications*	*Side-effects*
I/v	Children 2 mg/sq.m. body-surface Adults 1.4 mg/sq.m. body-surface	Lymphomas Leukaemias Wilm's tumour Lung cancer Breast cancer	Pregnancy To be given I/v.	Numbness and tingling sensation in hands and feet; Loss of hair.

15. Generic/Trade Names : *Vinblastin* VINBLASTIN (Khandelwal)

I/v	0.1 mg per kg body-wt initially, followed by 3 consecutive injections of 0.15 mg/kg body wt. at weekly intervals	Hodgkin's disease Lymphomas Cancers of the breast, utrine & bladder	Low WBC & Bacterial infections Low platelet count	Increased bleeding tendency; Increased risk of infection; Numbness and tingling sensation in hands and feet.

16. Generic/Trade Names : *Thiotepa* THIOTEPA (Cyanamid)

I/v	0.3 mg to 0.4 mg/kg body wt. at 1 to 4 weeks intervals.	Breast cancer Ovarian cancer	Lactating mothers; Liver disorder; Kidney disorder; Low WBC; Low platelet count	Increased risk of infection; Increased bleeding tendency; Nausea and vomiting; Infertility.

Glossary

Adenocarcinoma	A cancer starting in glandular tissue.
Adjuvant therapy	A secondary treatment which usually follows surgery and involves chemotherapy or radiation therapy.
Adrenalectomy	Removal of adrenal glands.
Adrenal glands	Two triangular endocrin e glands, each of which covers the upper surface of a kidney.
Aerosol	Tiniest particles of chemical suspended in air or gas inhaled from an inhaler.
Aflatoxin	A chemical derived from a fungus called Aspergillus, capable of causing liver cancer.
Alkalating agents	Chemicals that interfere with nucleic acid formation in the cells and thus prevent cells from multiplying, particularly in cases of cancer.
Amenorrhoea	Loss of normal menstruation.
Anaemia	Lack of red cells or haemoglobin in the blood.
Analgesics	Pain-relieving drugs.
Androgen	A male hormone.
Anti-metabolites	Anti-cancer drugs which interfere with the metabolism of cancer cells, and do not allow them to multiply.
Aromatic Amine	A chemical substance derived from petroleum products, said to be capable of causing cancer.

Ascitic fluid	Fluid that collects in the peritoneum in the abdomen. This may be due to tuberculosis, as well as other diseases including cancer.
Aspirate	Fluid sucked off with a syringe from anywhere in the body.
Benign	A term used to describe a tumour or tissue which is not cancerous, and which does not spread.
Bentu miners	Coal-miners of black race, belonging to a particular tribe in South Africa.
Benz(a) pyrene	A chemical substance produced after burning of petroleum products. It is said to be capable of producing cancer.
Bleeding time	Time taken after a slight cut in the skin stops bleeding. Low platelet count increases bleeding time.
Blood count	The number of red cells, white cells and platelets in a blood sample.
Bone marrow	Spongy tissue in the middle of bones that makes blood cells.
Bone marrow transplantation	Taking the bone marrow fluid from a donor and injecting it into the blood of a recepient. This is done in cases of leukaemia after selection of the donor. The bone marrow cells of a proper donor take root in the recipient and start producing new healthy line of blood cells.
Bronchoscopy	Examination of air passages with a metallic or flexible instrument called a bronchoscope.
Burkitt's lympoma	A lymphoma described by a European doctor named Burkitt while he was working in Africa.
Carcinogen	A substance that can cause or help cause cancer.
Carcinoma	A cancer that develops from cells called epithelial cells. These cells are present in

	the skin, lungs, glands, gastro-intestinal tract, and urinary tract. Cancers that develop in these sites are called carcinomas and are the commonest type of cancer.
Catecolamines	A special type of proteinous substance secreted by the adrenal glands and similar other cells in the body, which helps in regulating the functions of the body.
CAT scan	A computerized X-ray system that gives very clear pictures.
Cell	The cell is the basic unit of all living things or organisms.
Cervical smear	Smear made on a glass slide from the surface of the cervix of the uterus.
Chemotherapy	It is the treatment of cancer by means of drugs.
Clotting time	Time taken by the blood outside the body to change from a liquid state to a gelatinous one.
Clubbing of the finger nails	The nails over the fingers and also the toes become curved like the beak of a parrot. The terminal phalanx also becomes swollen and bulbous. This happens in many cases of lung cancer and some other non-cancer diseases also.
Colicky pain	Severe pain which increases in spasms.
Colon	It is a part of the large intestine.
Colonoscopy	The use of a flexible instrument to examine the entire large bowel.
Cyst	A closed cavity or sac that contains liquid or a semi-solid material.
Dibenz-anthracene	A chemical substance produced after burning of petroleum like products and also incomplete burning of tobacco. It is said to be capable of producing cancer.
Diethyl-stilbestrol	A compound of female sex hormone.

DNA	Deoxyribonucleic acid, the genetic material inside the nucleus of the cell which controls the cell's growth, division and function.
DLC	Different leukocyte count.
Duodenum	The first part of the small intestine.
Dysuria	Pain on passing urine.
Electro-encephalogram	Recording as waves, the minute quantity of electricity generated in the brain on its different surfaces.
Endocrine glands	Glands that secrete hormones into the bloodstream; examples are thyroid and pancreas.
Endoscopy	The use of a hollow instrument to examine the inside of different parts of the body.
Ependymoma	A cerebral or brain tumour derived from the glial (non-nervous) cells living the cavities of the brain.
Enzymes	Secretions of the special cells of the body, as for example of gastro-intestinal tract for digestion of food materials.
Epidedymitis	Inflammation of the epidedymus part of the testes.
Epidemiology	Study of geographical distribution of disease.
Epithelium	It is the lining that covers the internal and external surfaces of the body.
ESR	Erythrocyte (red blood cell) sedimentation rate. These cells in an unclotted blood settle at a particular rate in a particular time say, one hour. Rapid sedimentation rate indicates an inflammatory condition of the body or even a cancer.
Frozen section	A rapid way of examining a biopsy to see if it contains cancer; the result is available straightaway so that a suitable operation can be planned.

Gastro-enterology clinic	A clinic where diseases of the stomach and intestine are investigated and treated as a speciality.
Gastroscopy	Use of a flexible lighted instrument, which is swollowed to examine the inside of the stomach and the upper part of the small bowel.
Genetic	Inherited.
Gonadotrophin	A hormone normally secreted by the pituitary gland which stimulates the functions of the sex glands.
Granulocyto-paenia	Diminished counts of granulocyte (a type of white cells) in the blood.
Haematuria	Blood in the urine.
Hb	Haemoglobin.
Hepatitis-B virus	A virus transmitted through the blood, causing inflammation of the liver and its consequences.
Histology	Study of tissues to diagnose disease.
Hodgkin	An European doctor who first diagnosed and described the lymphoma now called after his name as Hodgkin's disease.
Hormone	A chemical substance secreted in the blood from the endocrine or hormonal glands, like insulin from pancreas or adrenaline from adrenal glands.
Hydrocele	Collection of fluid in the double-lined covering over the testes; the testes looks as if swollen.
Hypernephroma	A cancer of the kidney occurring in adults.
Hypertrophy	Increased growth of a tissue or an organ.
Hysterectomy	Removal of the uterus by surgical operation.
Ileostomy	An artificial opening between the small bowel (ileum) and the abdominal wall so that stool can be collected there in a bag.

Ileum	Last part of the small intestine in the abdomen.
Immuno-surveillance	Surveillance by lymphocytes and other cells in the blood, which destroy any cell or material which they consider as foreign and detrimental to the survival of the body.
In situ cancer	The earliest stage of a cancer where it is localized just where it started.
Laparotomy	An exploratory abdominal operation.
Laryngectomy	Surgical removal of the larynx.
Laryngoscopy	Examination of the larynx using a mirror.
Linear accelerator	A type of radiation therapy machine producing a very high energy radiation.
Lumber puncture	Puncture of the coverings of the spinal cord in the spinal column in the lumber area to collect a small quantity of cerebrospinal fluid for examination.
Lymph nodes	Nodules of tissue in the lymph channels that make lymphocytes and filter out unwanted substances.
Lymphatic system	Circulatory network of lymph-carrying vessels and the lymph nodes.
Malignant	A tumour which is cancerous and will spread with fatal results if not removed.
Mastectomy	An operation to surgically remove a breast having cancer.
Mediastinum	An area in the middle of the chest containing the heart, major blood vessels, etc.
Medulla	The inner region of any organ or tissue.
Menopause	Cessation of menstruation.
Mesothelioma	A type of cancer of the pleura.
Metastasis	Spread of cancer from one part of the body to another. The new area of cancer is a metastasis or secondary.
Mid-stream urine specimen	A specimen of urine taken in a sterile container a little after the start of mictu-

	rition, after having cleaned the local area. This is used for urine culture.
Morbidity	The symptoms or effects of a disease or its treatment.
Mortality rate	The death rate.
Mustard gas	A nervous system toxic gas, from which was derived the first anti-cancer drug, nitrogen mustard.
Mutation	A permanent change in the genetic material, DNA.
Narcotics	Drugs which can lead to unconsciousness.
Nepherectomy	Surgical removal of the kidney.
Nodule	A small swelling or aggregation of cells.
Oesophagus	Food pipe.
Ostomy	An artificial opening between an organ and the surface of the abdominal wall.
Palliative treatment	Treatment aimed at making a person feel better when cure is not possible.
Palpate	To feel by hand.
Pap-smear	A scrapping of cells from the cervix of the uterus for examination under a microscope.
Pathology	A branch of medicine concerned with the examination of diseased tissues.
Perfusion scanning of the lung	Making visible the channels in which the blood flows in the lungs. This is done by injecting into pulmonary circulation a radioactive substance which is then monitored.
Placebo	An inert substance used in controlled trials to see if a treatment is better than no treatment at all.
Platelets	Kind of cells in the blood that help it to clot.
Polycyclic aromatic hydrocarbons	Chemical substances related to petroleum products and also produced by incomplete burning of tabacco, said to be capable of causing cancer.

Polyp	A benign outgrowth of tissue.
Post-menopausal	Events that occur in the body after the cessation of the menstrual cycles, around the age of 45 years in women.
Primary cancer	A cancer present at the site in which it originated.
Prevalence	The total number of cases at any one time in a given area.
Prognosis	A prediction of the likely course of a disease.
Prophylactic	Treatment designed to prevent a disease.
Radical gastrectomy	A surgical operation in which the whole or a part of the stomach, and also the locally draining lymph glands are removed.
Radical mastectomy	An extensive surgical operation of the breast which removes some of the muscles of the chest wall also.
Radioactive substances	Substances that emit X-ray, etc.
Radioisotope	An atom of a metal having more or less electrons in it, which makes it unstable to exist in that state for long.
Radiosensitive	A cancer that shrinks or can be eradicated by a dose of radiation that is tolerated by nearby tissues.
RBC	Red blood cells
Relapse	The regrowth of a cancer after it has been removed or has responded to treatment.
Remission	Shrinkage of a tumour.
Retinoblastoma	A rare malignant tumour of the retina, occurring in infants. A retina in the light sensitive layer that lines the interior of the eye.
Roentgen	A German doctor who discovered X-rays in 1895.
Sarcoma	Cancers that develop in the body's supporting tissues like bone, cartilege, muscle, fat, tendons.

Solar radiation	Rays from the sun, some of which can cause cancer of the skin.
Stomatitis	Inflammation or soreness of the mouth.
Susruta	Ancient (600 BC) Indian surgeon who performed many skillful operations; *Susruta Samhita* is said to be composed by him.
Terminal care	Care of the patient when it is more or less certain that he will not survive much longer.
Tissue	A collection or mass of cells of one kind, such as of muscular tissue, nervous tissue, connective tissue, etc.
Thrombocytopeina	A reduction in the number of platelets in the blood.
TLC	Total leukocyte count.
Tomogram	X-ray of the chest taken with a special technique so that it shows the sharpest at a particular depth.
Tumour-marker	Biochemical substances produced by the tumour cells and poured in the blood, detection of which can help in diagnosing and following up the progress of the tumour.
Ultrasound	Sound waves of a frequency which are beyond hearing.
Urostomy	Artificial opening on the abdominal wall for passing out urine.
Ventilation scanning of the lung	Making visible the gas-containing parts of the lung. This is done by making the person inhale a radioactive gas, which can be monitored from over the lung.

Also in Orient Paperbacks

High Blood Pressure: Causes, Prevention & Treatment
Dr Krishan Gupta, MD, FRCP, FACP

A practical guide for the prevention and control of high blood pressure and its complications; an invaluable source of information to help you stay healthy and live longer.

High Blood Cholesterol: Causes, Prevention & Treatment
Dr Krishan Gupta, MD, FRCP, FACP

High Blood Cholesterol, a major cause of heart attacks, can be prevented, controlled and reversed; this life-extending book tells you how.

'If you have high cholesterol levels, get hold of this book.'

Times of India

Arthritis: Causes, Prevention & Treatment
Ada P. Kahn, MPH

'... simple and easy-to-understand.'

Deccan Herald

Diabetes: Causes, Prevention & Treatment
Ada P. Kahn, MPH

'... of great help to those suffering from diabetes ... to keep it under control.'

Dr M.C. Srivastava Diabetic Self-Care Foundation, India

Neck Pain: Causes, Prevention & Treatment
Dr Arthur Winter, MD, FICS and Ruth Winter, MS

A straight talking, no-nonsense, practical guide to treating and preventing neck pain.